AF182412

Teamwork in Healthcare

Edited by Michael S. Firstenberg
and Stanislaw P. Stawicki

Published in London, United Kingdom

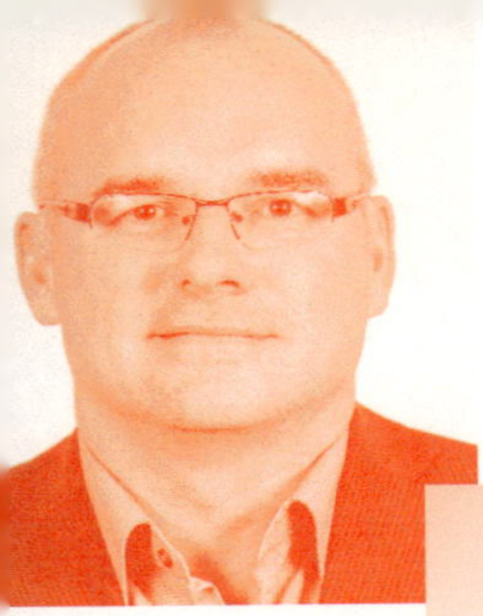
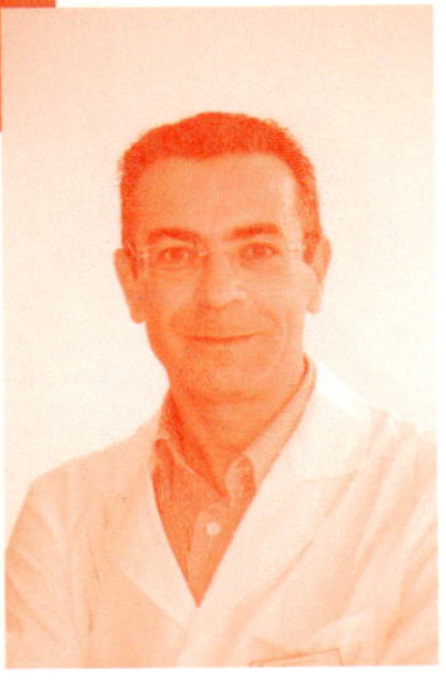
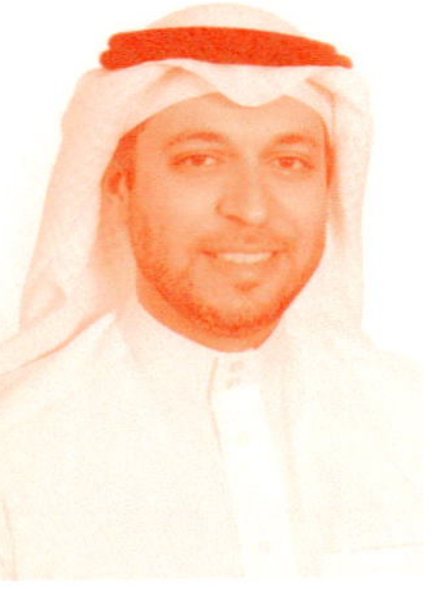
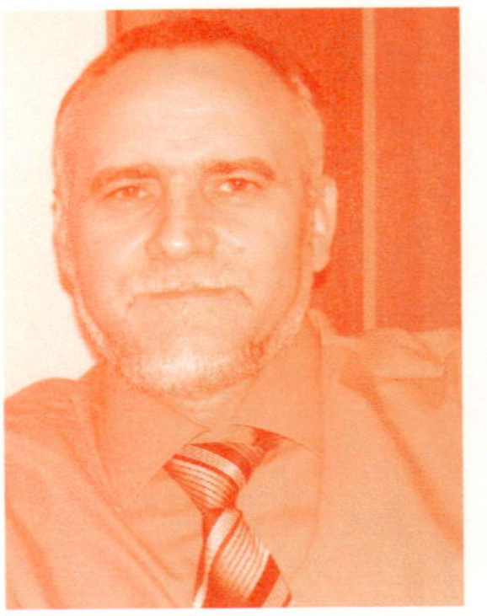
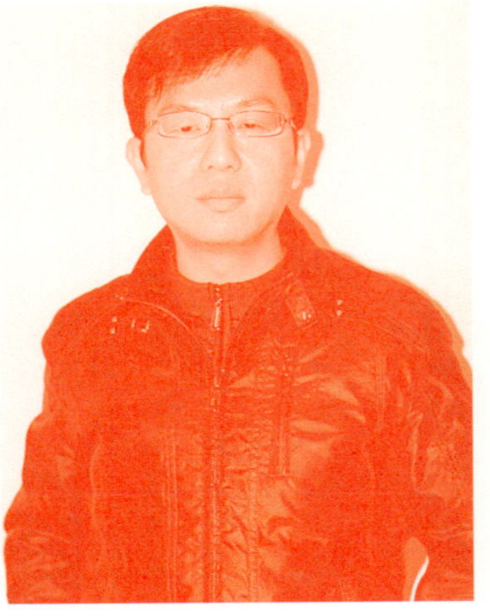
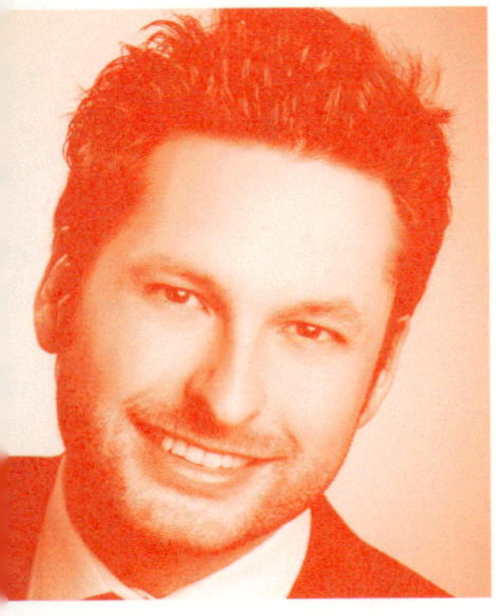
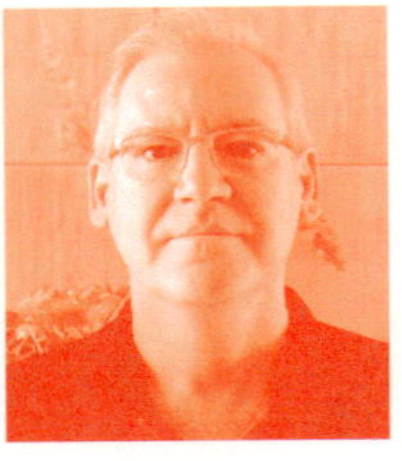

IntechOpen

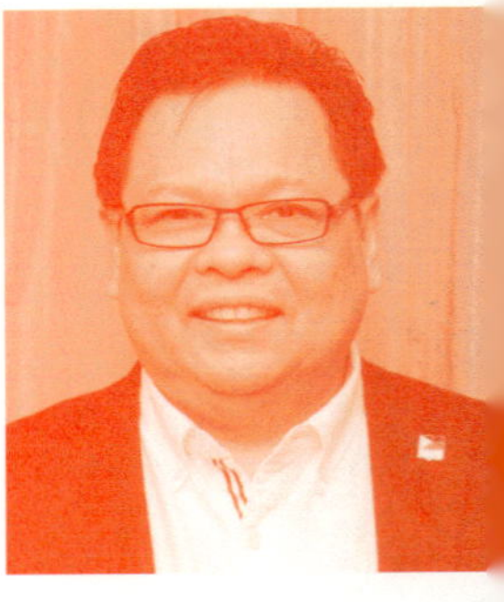
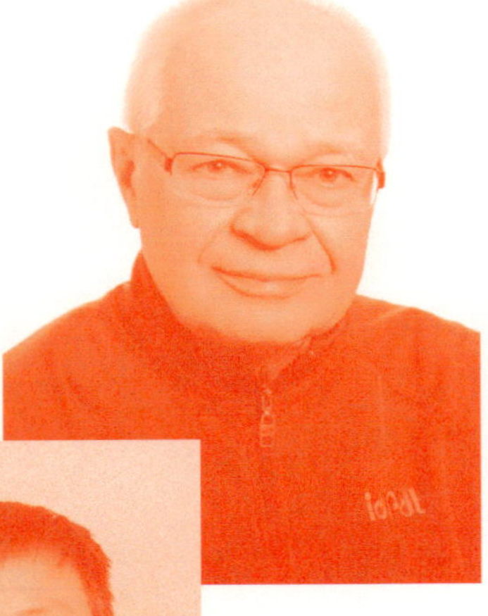
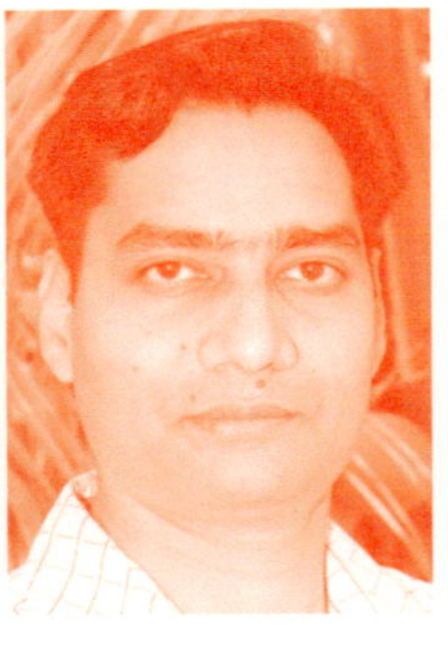
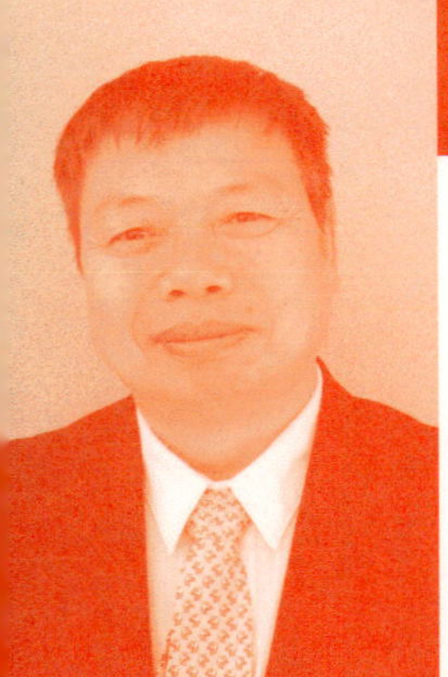
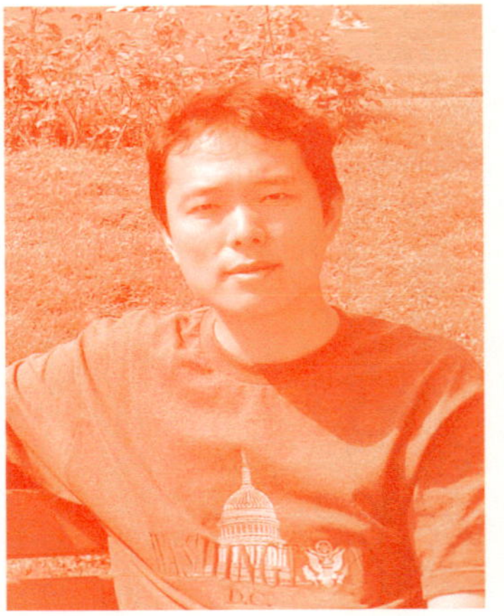
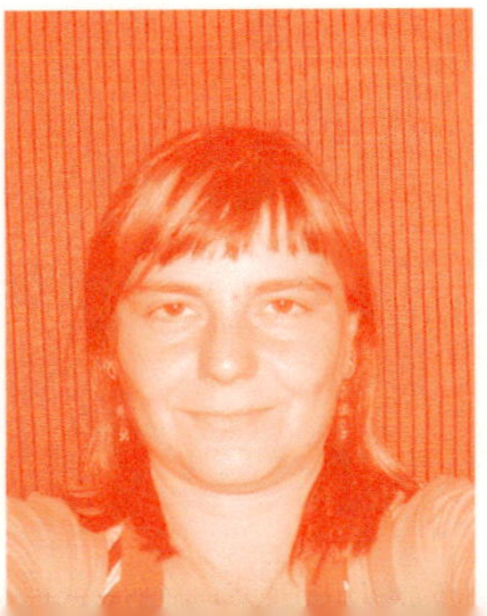

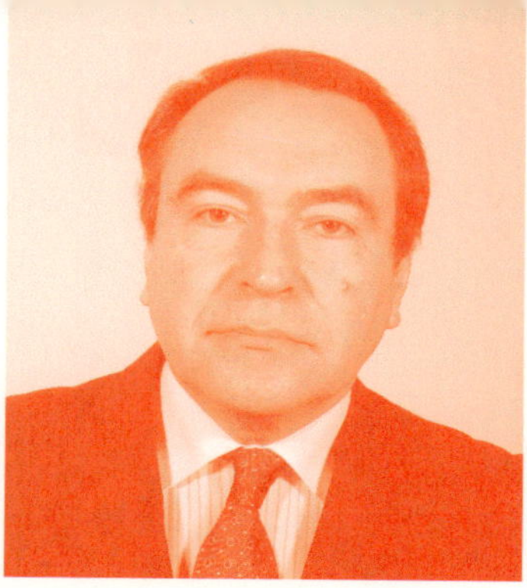
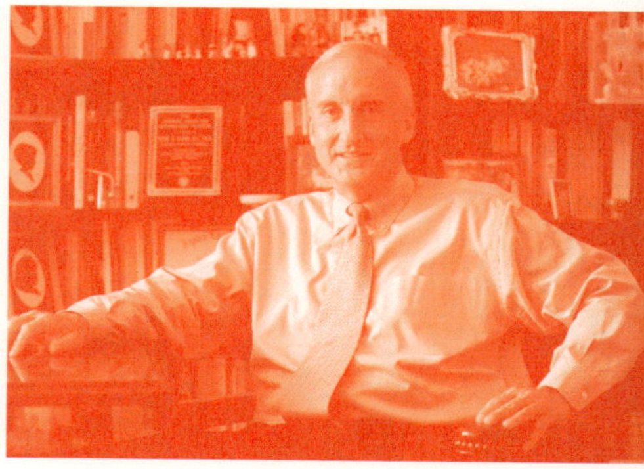
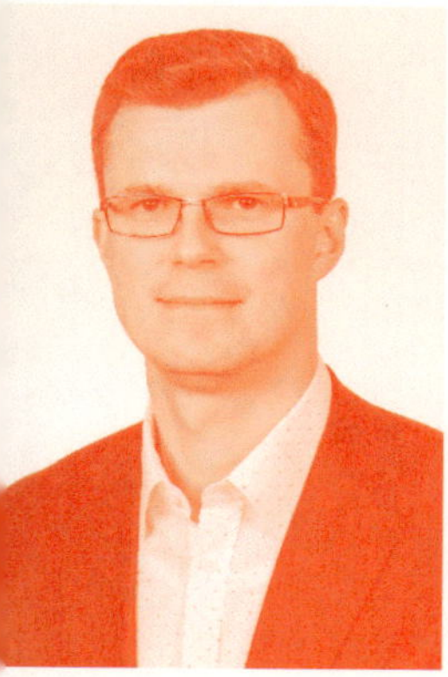
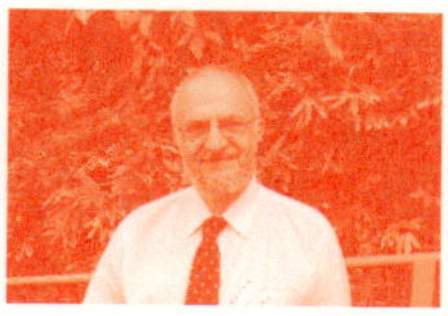
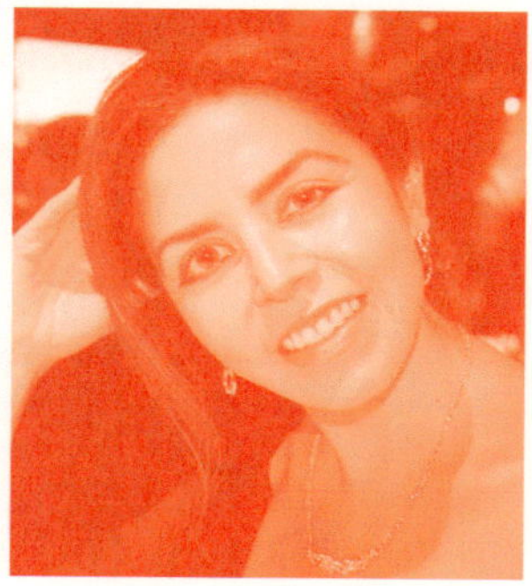

Supporting open minds since 2005

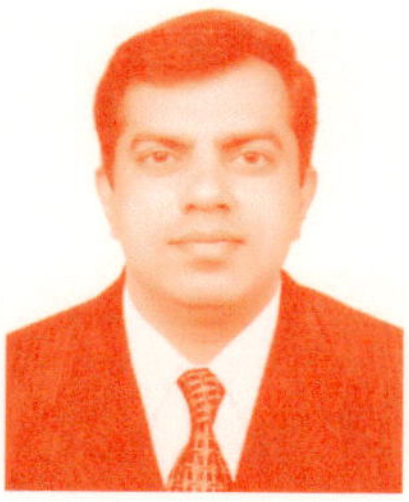
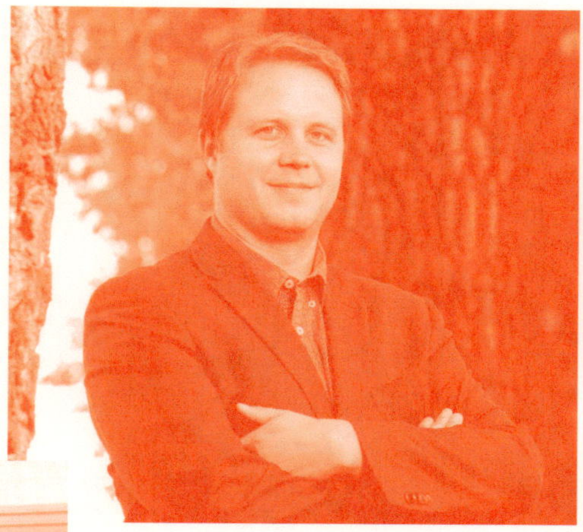
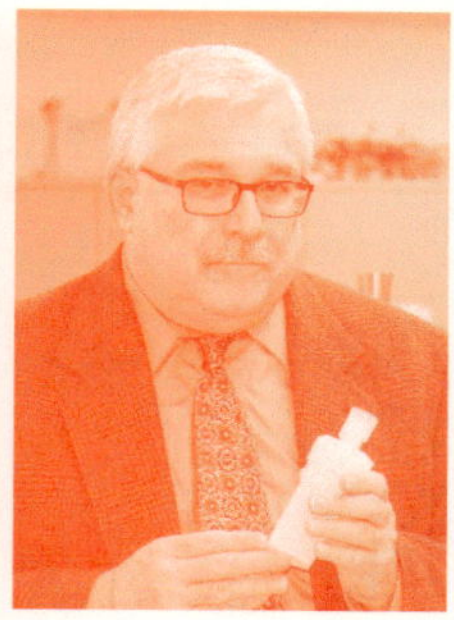
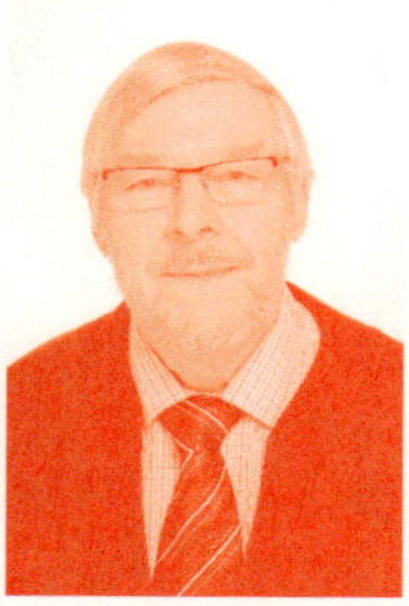
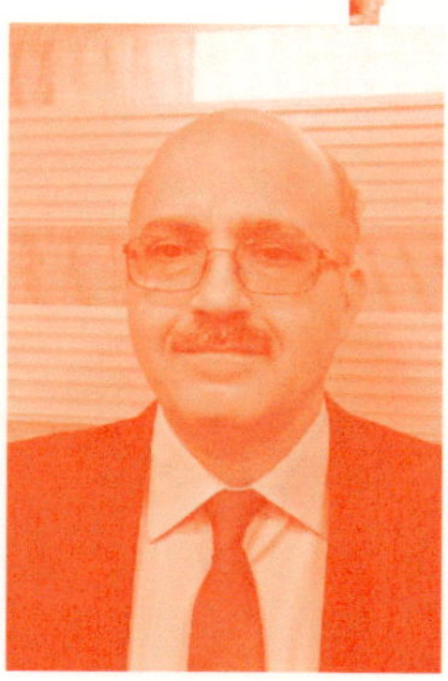
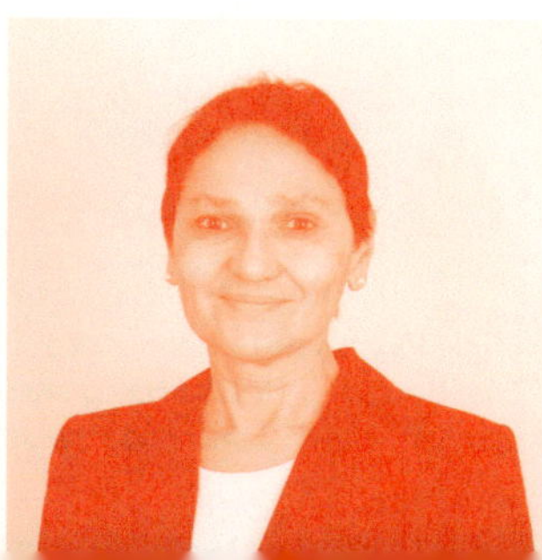
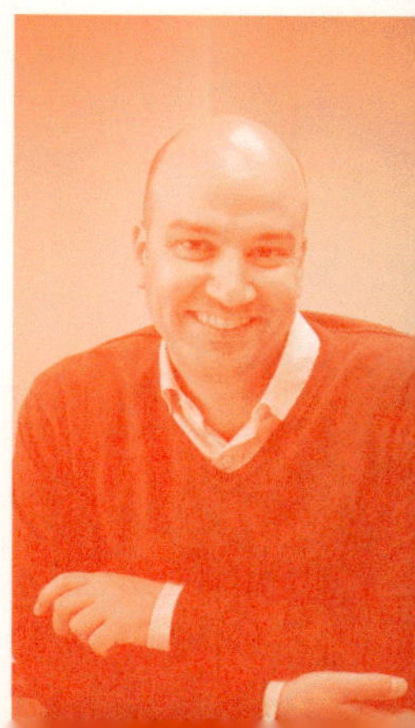

Teamwork in Healthcare
http://dx.doi.org/10.5772/intechopen.87354
Edited by Michael S. Firstenberg and Stanislaw P. Stawicki

Contributors
Gabor Xantus, Laszlo Zavori, Giovanni Barbanti Brodano, Cristiana Griffoni, Alessandro Gasbarrini, Alessandro Ricci, Sandra Giannone, Francesca Elena Daniela Ghisi, Giulio Nittari, Iolanda Grappasonni, Stefania Scuri, Fabio Petrelli, Getu Gamo Sagaro, Nikolai Ramadanov, Nemandra Sandiford, You Chen, Maria Joelle, Merce Mach, Ceferí Soler-Vicente, António C. M. Abrantes, Azzadin Mahmod, Saadia Khuder, Stanislaw P. Stawicki, Michael S. Firstenberg, Israel Zighelboim, Nicholas Taylor, Farhad Sholevar, Vasfiye Bayram Değer, Konrad Wronka

© The Editor(s) and the Author(s) 2021
The rights of the editor(s) and the author(s) have been asserted in accordance with the Copyright, Designs and Patents Act 1988. All rights to the book as a whole are reserved by INTECHOPEN LIMITED. The book as a whole (compilation) cannot be reproduced, distributed or used for commercial or non-commercial purposes without INTECHOPEN LIMITED's written permission. Enquiries concerning the use of the book should be directed to INTECHOPEN LIMITED rights and permissions department (permissions@intechopen.com).
Violations are liable to prosecution under the governing Copyright Law.

CC BY

Individual chapters of this publication are distributed under the terms of the Creative Commons Attribution 3.0 Unported License which permits commercial use, distribution and reproduction of the individual chapters, provided the original author(s) and source publication are appropriately acknowledged. If so indicated, certain images may not be included under the Creative Commons license. In such cases users will need to obtain permission from the license holder to reproduce the material. More details and guidelines concerning content reuse and adaptation can be found at http://www.intechopen.com/copyright-policy.html.

Notice
Statements and opinions expressed in the chapters are these of the individual contributors and not necessarily those of the editors or publisher. No responsibility is accepted for the accuracy of information contained in the published chapters. The publisher assumes no responsibility for any damage or injury to persons or property arising out of the use of any materials, instructions, methods or ideas contained in the book.

First published in London, United Kingdom, 2021 by IntechOpen
IntechOpen is the global imprint of INTECHOPEN LIMITED, registered in England and Wales, registration number: 11086078, 5 Princes Gate Court, London, SW7 2QJ, United Kingdom
Printed in Croatia

British Library Cataloguing-in-Publication Data
A catalogue record for this book is available from the British Library

Additional hard and PDF copies can be obtained from orders@intechopen.com

Teamwork in Healthcare
Edited by Michael S. Firstenberg and Stanislaw P. Stawicki
p. cm.
Print ISBN 978-1-83881-028-3
Online ISBN 978-1-83881-029-0
eBook (PDF) ISBN 978-1-83881-030-6

For EU product safety concerns:
IN TECH d.o.o., Prolaz Marije Krucifikse Kozulić 3, 51000 Rijeka, Croatia, info@intechopen.com or visit our website at intechopen.com.

We are IntechOpen, the world's leading publisher of Open Access books

Built by scientists, for scientists

5,200+
Open access books available

129,000+
International authors and editors

155M+
Downloads

156
Countries delivered to

Our authors are among the
Top 1%
most cited scientists

12.2%
Contributors from top 500 universities

WEB OF SCIENCE™

Selection of our books indexed in the Book Citation Index in Web of Science™ Core Collection (BKCI)

Interested in publishing with us?
Contact book.department@intechopen.com

Numbers displayed above are based on latest data collected.
For more information visit www.intechopen.com

Meet the editors

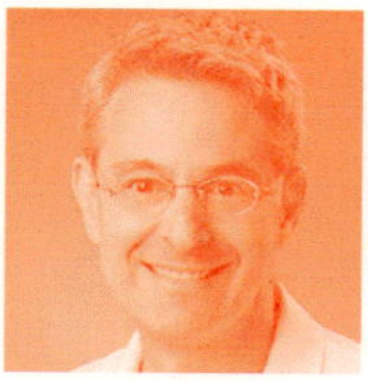

Dr. Michael S. Firstenberg is a board-certified thoracic surgeon. He is the current Director of Research and Special Projects for the William Novick Global Cardiac Alliance. Previously, he was Chief of Cardiothoracic and Vascular Surgery at the Medical Center of Aurora and Rose Hospitals. He currently holds appointments in the Colleges of Medicine and Graduate Studies at Northeast Ohio Medical University. He attended Case Western Reserve University Medical School, received his General Surgery training at University Hospitals in Cleveland, and completed fellowships at Ohio State University (Thoracic Surgery) and the Cleveland Clinic (Surgical Heart Failure). He is an active member of the Society of Thoracic Surgeons (STS), the American Association of Thoracic Surgeons (AATS), the American College of Cardiology (ACC), and the American College of Academic International Medicine (ACAIM), for which he is a founding fellow and president-elect. He currently serves on several professional society committees. He is the author of more than 200 peer-reviewed manuscripts, abstracts, and book chapters. He has edited several textbooks on topics ranging from medical leadership, patient safety, endocarditis, and extra-corporeal membrane oxygenation, all of which include topics that he has lectured on worldwide.

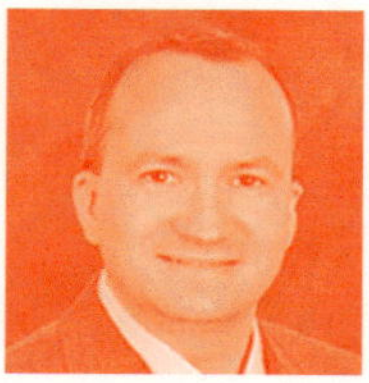

Dr. Stanislaw P. Stawicki is Professor of Surgery and Chair, Department of Research and Innovation, St. Luke's University Health Network, Bethlehem, Pennsylvania. A specialist in General Surgery, Surgical Critical Care, and Neurocritical Care, Dr. Stawicki has co-authored more than 640 scholarly works, including more than twenty books. In addition to national and international medical leadership roles, he is a member of numerous editorial boards. His areas of expertise include blockchain technology, patient safety, academic leadership, mentorship, trauma/critical care, and sonography.

Contents

Preface

One of the most significant advances in patient care is the recognition that high-quality healthcare, as defined by optimal outcomes achieved safely, in a timely and efficient manner, is best delivered by teams working together. The concept of teamwork in healthcare, as emphasized in this text, is critical at all levels – from the bedside of the patient up to all tiers of administrative support. Critical to our understanding of the role of teams is the recognition that there is an inherent advantage of groups working together in increasingly complex settings. Consequently, it must be emphasized that teams must be able to function within a structure that is guided by multi-disciplinary approaches, excellent communication, and a clear focus on high-quality and successful patient outcomes. Important aspects of teams and teamwork in healthcare include the assurance that teams are properly defined with regards to membership, roles, responsibilities, and group objectives that can be measured. Accomplishing such objectives is not always easy – especially since there must be "buy-in" toward the overall structure and function at all levels. Champions, typically physicians and their administrative support, are crucial to success.

As several chapters in this text emphasize, it is important that teams, once defined, have clear objectives and goals. With individual roles, responsibilities, and accountability defined, an entire group (and interfacing groups) can work together toward achieving common goals by taking full advantage of the strengths of the group working both as individuals and jointly while mitigating potential weakness and deficiencies inherent to more individualistic approaches. Such successes should be objectively measured, shared, and celebrated, focusing on improved outcomes (e.g., survival, length of stay, costs, patient/family satisfaction, etc.).

Many of the concepts discussed in this volume are constantly evolving. Because of this, each chapter serves as a basic foundation to encourage the reader to explore the references and actively engage in discovering (and contributing to) the latest advances in the healthcare "team science." On behalf of the entire editorial team, we would like to thank all the authors for their hard work, dedication, and outstanding contributions to this project. We also appreciate the interest of the readers in providing a forum for discussion of these dynamic, rapidly evolving, and complex topics.

Michael S. Firstenberg, MD FACC FAIM
William Novick Global Cardiac Alliance,
United States of America

Stanislaw P. Stawicki, MD MBA FACS FAIM
St. Luke's University Health Network,
United States of America

Section 1

Foundations in Teamwork

Chapter 1

Introductory Chapter: Teams in Healthcare - A Voyage from 'Nice to Have' to 'the Way to Go'

Nicholas Taylor, Israel Zighelboim, Farhad Sholevar, Stanislaw P. Stawicki and Michael S. Firstenberg

1. Introduction

Modern healthcare is characterized by the growing embrace of multidisciplinary, team-based approaches. This transformation is happening for a good reason. Because the degree of complexity across our health systems may exceed the effective operational capacity of a single provider, increasing reliance on healthcare teams, processes, and workflows is becoming a necessity [1, 2]. Despite the near universal deployment of health information technology, the overall growth in systemic complexity continues to outpace our attempts to address it [3, 4]. The ability to adapt and evolve also plays an essential role in achieving programmatic success [5].

The current team-based approach to healthcare originated in the 1990's in an attempt to enhance the performance, quality and safety of care delivery [6–8]. Through a series of incremental changes and reforms, significant improvements have been made over time, but the healthcare industry is still far from the safety, quality, and performance records achieved by our counterparts in financial and air transportation sectors [9]. Currently, a significant portion of the overall effort in this area revolves around reinforcing team-based approaches, including the incorporation of continuous quality and performance improvement initiatives into existing, multidisciplinary paradigms across a broad range of care delivery settings [7, 10, 11].

2. How do teams make healthcare better?

Although there is something to be said about the expression, "the whole is greater than the sum of the parts," our current understanding of full benefits of a 'healthcare team' continues to be relatively limited [12–15]. The very presence of a 'team' does not inherently equate to enhanced levels of quality or safety. Yet there clearly is an evolving science dedicated to learning more and refining our approach to healthcare team effectiveness [16–18]. As a result, a number of key characteristics associated with optimal team performance have been proposed [15, 19, 20]. We will discuss them in this section.

Although this may be an 'obvious' statement, healthcare teams should be able to maintain high levels of functioning at all times [19]. More granular considerations in this area include constant focus on coordination, emphasis on responsibility, and the full commitment to open and honest communication (even if the latter exposes

IntechOpen

one's lack of specific/granular patient care knowledge) [19]. Some variability and customization of the overall team approach should be permitted, even encouraged, based on the setting, situation, or available resources. This provides the necessary flexibility to accomplish a much broader range (and types) of tasks. Beyond these fundamental values, effective healthcare teams must be highly skilled in their 'teamwork ability' – inclusive of dedicated education about interdisciplinary, non-hierarchical, consensus-based approaches [21]. In the perfect world, application of the above principles results in seamless delivery of care, with minimal or no biases, without silos, using data-driven, patient centered approaches [22, 23].

Unfortunately, a major assumption in the concept of adopting "team-based healthcare" is that "individuals" inherently desire to be part of a "team." However, as it is well known, such desire is not universal. While it may sound like a rhetorical question when asking, "Why healthcare providers would not want to be engaged in such an evolution?" – It is important to explore some of the potential motivating factors that contribute to the development of "team-based" care. Unfortunately, some of these factors involve certain key harsh realities that strongly influence healthcare providers. Everyone inherently claims that they "want what is best for the patient" – but such a concept is difficult to comprehensively and universally define, especially in the setting in which "individuals" might not want to be part of a "team" for several reasons:

1. They do not feel that their participation in a team (i.e., morning multi-disciplinary rounds) is helpful to the overall care of the patient.

2. They may not want to participate because they do not find the structure and function of the team as being compatible with their daily work-flow, or inherently useful in the context of their multiple competing obligations.

3. Financial (or professional) motives and/or agendas may not be compatible with the team-based culture. This is a consideration that is particularly applicable in various "pay-for-service" healthcare models in which team-based care might not inherently be in everyone's best financial interest. Such situations are becoming more common when team activities – such as patient-care conferences (e.g., "tumor boards" or "heart team meetings") – might be best for discussing patient care plans, but do not generate any immediate financial opportunities for participants while diminishing the latter due to built-in time constraints.

4. Team-based care models are not structured in a way to optimize the common goals – especially in a manner that is respectful of the expertise and time commitments of all participating stakeholders.

5. Leadership (or senior administrators) may not inherently support the concept and applications of team-based approaches. Potential administrative road-blocks can be subtle, such as limiting resources available for the required support staff or not supporting (publicly or privately) the team goals or individual champions.

While there are many reasons why team-based care models either work or do not work – the fundamental key or barrier to success is engagement, support, enthusiasm, and expertise, or lack thereof, by leaders, champions, and those who believe that team-based care is fundamentally better in terms of patient outcomes. This should be contrasted against individuals who may be "siloed" in their inflexible, individualistic, and potentially self-gain motivated models.

3. Healthcare teams and evidence-based practice

The team-based setting is the optimal environment for the implementation of evidence-based practice. Inherent to the team approach in healthcare is the presence of ample cross-checks, safety protocols, and the ability to verify clinical plans via a consensus mechanism [24, 25]. This, in turn, helps facilitate the application of evidence-base practice, which appears to be both safer and relatively free of personal biases and/or opinions [8, 26]. Moreover, 'team healthcare' environment also provides an excellent substrate for determining that a given protocol or clinical pathway does not work, thus prompting constructive changes that tend to be evidence-based and systematic in nature [10]. Again, success is based upon the participation of champions, leadership support at all levels, and the recognition that such paradigm shifts within a 'culture of behaviors' are better for all aspects of the patient care, including both experiences and outcomes – and not just for individuals who continue to advocate that "the old ways," which might have worked to some degree in the past, are still acceptable across modern healthcare delivery platforms [7, 14, 24, 27].

4. Team approaches help reduce burnout

In addition to the patient-specific benefits of team-based healthcare, growing amount of data point toward tangible provider benefits of team-based approaches, including reduction in burnout [28]. It has been suggested that implementation of certain structural changes, such as fostering communication between team members and cultivating a sense of teamwork and job control are very effective in reducing provider burnout [29]. An important factor in this general approach is the ability of teammates to motivate each other and to encourage accountability for key behaviors, such as regular physical exercise and gym attendance [30]. As with many other areas that depend on highly functioning teams (e.g., airline crews or professional sports), the ability of a team to function effectively and efficiently is the overarching priority, even when a particular team member is temporarily underperforming or sidelined. More complex performance issues, including disruptive team member behaviors, can also be addressed in a professional and collaborative manner with the common team goals maintained as a priority [31, 32].

5. Teams as agents of positive institutional change

Healthcare teams contribute tremendously to structural institutional and systemic changes. In aggregate, such changes tend to occur more gradually and are typically due to consensus-building mechanisms inherent to team approaches. The resulting action plans, in general, tend to be both constructive and more readily embraced by key stakeholders.

Healthcare settings require fluid, coordinated and effective work of various highly integrated teams across the continuum of care. Due to the complex nature and integrated character of the industry, effective "teaming" in healthcare must expand across organizational boundaries [33]. The effective delivery of health services typically requires the integration of special skills, equipment and care that must often be provided around the clock at variable locations. Additionally, the historic hierarchy encountered in hospitals generates status differences which may potentially contribute to misunderstanding, hesitation to communicate any disagreement, as well as difficulty in pointing out errors and opportunities [15, 34–36]. Finally, patients with complex or chronic diseases interact with multiple levels of a cumbersome health care delivery system (inpatient and outpatient settings, laboratories, imaging centers, etc). This, in turn, creates multiple opportunities for team-based paradigms to facilitate more unified, patient-centered approaches [37].

Deployment of effective "teaming" represents a valuable tool to exert positive institutional change. In doing so it is critical to reframe goals and objectives. Tasks in health care should be framed in a way that allows each team member to focus on the ultimate goal beyond the current intervention – the individual patient outcome. Such approach encourages team members to go beyond their limited area of expertise in order to seek and promote other beneficial interventions or services. In addition, effective teaming requires the use of safety as the quintessential bar to measure team effectiveness. In doing so, the team approach becomes the instrument to break through hierarchical barriers. At the end of the day, every member of the team will agree that providing safe care is a must. It is imperative to create structures and methodologies that foster open communication and trust. Tools such as the SBAR method (situation, background, assessment and recommendation) or the Team STEPPS approach are relatively easy to deploy and track [7, 15, 18, 38, 39].

A comprehensive transformation toward more widespread reliance on team approaches across our healthcare systems will help promote dependability, establish and/or strengthen mutual trust, foster open communication, and enhance collaboration among both individuals and teams. The result commonly translates into improved quality and safety, cost-effectiveness and importantly improved team members' satisfaction. All of the above are key elements for the success of any health care organization.

6. Teams versus committees versus task-forces

Understanding the differences between teams, task forces, and committees can help further solidify the importance of a collaborative environment with focused goals [40, 41]. While there are a variety of definitions of each, in the context of healthcare, there are certain key differences between the 3 groups [42–44]. Below we summarize the definitions that, in the Editors' opinion, are most applicable to this current book.

6.1 Teams

1. Typically comprise of individuals linked together for a common purpose;

2. There is a shared leadership model (e.g., collaboration to achieve a specific task);

3. Members often have complementary skills and are encouraged to function as a group;

4. Team members share a common goal or purpose, with mutual accountability [45].

6.2 Committees

1. Typically consist of individuals who are selected to perform a specific function on behalf of a larger group;

2. Committee is technically a structured organizational system – often with agenda, bylaws, and strong leadership;

3. Finally, committees may not have a fixed endpoint or goal, and may be structured to delegate specific tasks to smaller groups (e.g., subcommittees) [46, 47].

6.3 Task forces

1. These are typically small groups with densely concentrated content expertise, usually brought together to focus on a specific goal;

2. Task forces are usually organized on an "as needed basis" – potentially in response to an event;

3. Although there may be limited objective resources to achieve a highly specific goal, task forces are often asked to make recommendations to a Committee before any final changes are executed [48, 49].

It is important to remember that, as in many other functional organizational areas, there are overlaps in structure and function among these different groups. At the same time, each type of team/group participation is needed – for different purposes as noted above – within an organization to ensure stability and objective preemptive or responsive problem solving. Consequently, careful planning and balancing of goals, roles, and priorities is required.

7. Pitfalls of teams and team-based approaches

One of the greatest pitfalls of teams and team-based approaches is the ever-present danger of 'groupthink' [50]. Groupthink can be defined as the presence of social conformity within a group tasked with making a collective decision [51]. When analyzed retrospectively, group decisions based on 'groupthink' are often influenced by the 'single loudest voice' or authority within the group, with the apparent absence of critical thinking and/or the 'fortitude to question' exhibited by individual members of that group [50, 52]. At a much deeper level, 'groupthink' is a symptom of poor leadership, where the leader (whether positionally assigned or not) may not challenge or empower his or her team sufficiently enough to effectively question the course of the discussion around the prevailing group sentiment [53–56]. Hence, it is imperative that team leadership recognizes the potential for such disruptive forces and – as a sign of strength and wisdom – actively monitors for (and attenuates) the impact of factors and/or individuals capable of "inducing groupthink." Conceptually, mitigating against "groupthink" sounds easy, but in practice it can be extremely difficult – if not impossible – when the loudest voice is often the one with the greatest perceived influence [57, 58]. Such issues are unfortunately not uncommon in healthcare when significant financial and non-financial agendas might be directly linked to individuals or groups who may then be compelled to act in a manner that might be in their best interest, but not in the interest of the larger group or team. Such situations can be extremely difficult to manage or control – and ultimately require a significant disruptive event (like an institutional financial crisis or exodus of talent) or systemic change.

8. Limitations to team approaches

As the reader embarks on exploring this book, it must be emphasized that certain activities and/or circumstances do not lend themselves to team approaches.

Although this will not be the focus of this edited collection, we want the reader to be aware of those important limitations to team-based approaches. For example, there exists a balance between team-based and non-team-based management in the area of execution capability [59].

It is also important to know when and how to limit team sizes, especially when specific types of tasks or mission-critical endeavors demand such limited approach. In medicine, teams are ubiquitous. There are highly diversified health-care teams inclusive of medical/nursing students, residents, nurses, physicians, case managers, physical/occupational therapists and consulting physicians/teams. Not infrequently, the more complex the patient, the larger the care team tends to grow. At many institutions, there are annual celebrations of Trauma Systems, highlighting the health-care journey of trauma/critical care patients. During such celebrations, the entire health-care team caring for critically injured patients is gradually, person-by-person, brought on stage, with upwards of 100 people responsible for the successful door-to-door care involving each individual trauma survivor [60].

Clearly, utilizing teams to leverage different areas of clinical expertise is necessary. Although these large teams are good at solving problems, the larger the team, the more likely communication failures can occur, increasing the aggregate risk of medical errors [61–63]. Smaller teams, on the other hand, have been shown to be more disruptive and innovative and will be more likely to identify new problems for the larger team to solve [64]. Across all aspects of patient care, limiting team size can reduce some of the less savory aspects of a team approach like conformity bias and social loafing [65]. Ultimately, it is important to select the most optimal team for the job [66] and limit team size when high-impact communication and innovation are critical. Larger teams can then be layered over the smaller teams to use the "wisdom of crowds" and improve decision making [65]. Regardless of team size, it is important to continue to study the different team-based approaches to determine whether we are succeeding in improving patient/system outcomes.

9. Conclusions

Modern healthcare is firmly set on its quest toward better, safer, more efficient, high quality patient care delivery. A critical part of this decades-long transition is the gradual realization that teamwork, based on multidisciplinary, data-driven, evidence-based, patient-centric approaches, is now 'the way to go' and much more than a 'good to have' luxury. This book is dedicated to the exploration of concepts critical to our better understanding of the dynamically evolving area of team-based healthcare.

Author details

Nicholas Taylor[1], Israel Zighelboim[1], Farhad Sholevar[2], Stanislaw P. Stawicki[3] and Michael S. Firstenberg[4*]

1 Department of Obstetrics and Gynecology, St. Luke's University Health Network, Bethlehem, Pennsylvania, USA

2 Department of Psychiatry, St. Luke's University Health Network, Bethlehem, Pennsylvania, USA

3 Department of Research and Innovation, St. Luke's University Health Network, Bethlehem, Pennsylvania, USA

4 William Novick Cardiac Alliance, Memphis, TN, USA

*Address all correspondence to: msfirst@gmail.com

IntechOpen

© 2021 The Author(s). Licensee IntechOpen. This chapter is distributed under the terms of the Creative Commons Attribution License (http://creativecommons.org/licenses/by/3.0), which permits unrestricted use, distribution, and reproduction in any medium, provided the original work is properly cited.

References

[1] Baker, D.P., R. Day, and E. Salas, *Teamwork as an essential component of high-reliability organizations.* Health services research, 2006. **41**(4p2): p. 1576-1598.

[2] Rosen, M.A., et al., *Teamwork in healthcare: Key discoveries enabling safer, high-quality care.* American Psychologist, 2018. **73**(4): p. 433.

[3] Tidd, J. and J.R. Bessant, *Managing innovation: integrating technological, market and organizational change*. 2018: John Wiley & Sons.

[4] Kellermann, A.L. and S.S. Jones, *What it will take to achieve the as-yet-unfulfilled promises of health information technology.* Health affairs, 2013. **32**(1): p. 63-68.

[5] Pype, P., et al., *Healthcare teams as complex adaptive systems: understanding team behaviour through team members' perception of interpersonal interaction.* BMC health services research, 2018. **18**(1): p. 570.

[6] Stawicki, S., *Fundamentals of patient safety in medicine and surgery*. 2015: Wolters kluwer india Pvt Ltd.

[7] Tolentino, J.C., et al., *Introductory chapter: Developing patient safety champions.* Vignettes in Patient Safety, 2018. **2**: p. 1-23.

[8] Stawicki, S.P. and M.S. Firstenberg, *Introductory chapter: The decades long quest continues toward better, safer healthcare systems.* Vignettes in Patient Safety, 2017. **1**: p. 1.

[9] Portner, M., et al., *Learning from others: Examples from air transportation and industrial realms.* Stawicki S et al. Fundamentals of Patient Safety in Medicine and Surgery. New Delhi: Wolters Kluwer Health (India) Pvt Ltd, 2014.

[10] Saeed, M., et al., *Fact versus conjecture: Exploring levels of evidence in the context of patient safety and care quality*, in *Vignettes in Patient Safety-Volume 3*. 2018, IntechOpen.

[11] Gracias, V.H., et al., *Critical care nurse practitioners improve compliance with clinical practice guidelines in "semiclosed" surgical intensive care unit.* Journal of Nursing Care Quality, 2008. **23**(4): p. 338-344.

[12] Makadok, R., *Doing the right thing and knowing the right thing to do: Why the whole is greater than the sum of the parts.* Strategic Management Journal, 2003. **24**(10): p. 1043-1055.

[13] Salas, E. and M.A. Rosen, *Building high reliability teams: progress and some reflections on teamwork training.* BMJ quality & safety, 2013. **22**(5): p. 369-373.

[14] Green, A., S.P. Stawicki, and M.S. Firstenberg, *Introductory Chapter: Medical Error and Associated Harm-The The Critical Role of Team Communication and Coordination*, in *Vignettes in Patient Safety-Volume 3*. 2018, IntechOpen.

[15] Brathwaite, S., et al., *Teaching Characteristics and Fostering for Patient Leadership Safety.* Fundamentals of Patient Safety in Medicine and Surgery, 2015: p. 153.

[16] Thomas, E.J., *Improving teamwork in healthcare: current approaches and the path forward.* BMJ quality & safety, 2011. **20**(8): p. 647-650.

[17] Wilson, K.A., et al., *Promoting health care safety through training high reliability teams.* BMJ quality & safety, 2005. **14**(4): p. 303-309.

[18] Papadimos, T.J. and S.P. Stawicki, *Chapter 32: Role of Prospective Approaches in Patient Safety and Patient Safety Research.* Fundamentals

of Patient Safety in Medicine and Surgery, 2015: p. 309.

[19] Mitchell, P., et al., *Core principles & values of effective team-based health care.* NAM Perspectives, 2012.

[20] Latchana, N., J.R. Peck, and S.P. Stawicki, *How and Why Things Go Wrong: The Art of Unbiased Understanding.* Fundamentals of Patient Safety in Medicine and Surgery, 2015: p. 77.

[21] Boon, H., et al., *From parallel practice to integrative health care: a conceptual framework.* BMC health services research, 2004. **4**(1): p. 15.

[22] Erickson, S.M., et al., *Envisioning a Better US Health Care System for All: Health Care Delivery and Payment System Reforms.* Annals of internal medicine, 2020. **172**(2_Supplement): p. S33-S49.

[23] Ochoa, J.G.D. and F. Weil, *From personalization to patient centered systems toxicology and pharmacology.* Computational Toxicology, 2019. **11**: p. 14-22.

[24] Stawicki, S. and A. Gerlach, *Polypharmacy and medication errors: Stop, listen, look, and analyze.* Opus, 2009. **12**: p. 6-10.

[25] Smith, E., et al., *Surgical safety checklist: Productive, nondisruptive, and the" right thing to do".* Journal of postgraduate medicine, 2015. **61**(3): p. 214.

[26] Stevens, K., *The impact of evidence-based practice in nursing and the next big ideas.* The Online Journal of Issues in Nursing, 2013. **18**(2).

[27] Bach, J.A., et al., *The right team at the right time–Multidisciplinary approach to multi-trauma patient with orthopedic injuries.* International journal of critical illness and injury science, 2017. **7**(1): p. 32.

[28] Smith, C.D., et al., *Implementing optimal team-based care to reduce clinician burnout.* NAM Perspectives, 2018.

[29] Linzer, M., et al., *A cluster randomized trial of interventions to improve work conditions and clinician burnout in primary care: results from the Healthy Work Place (HWP) study.* Journal of general internal medicine, 2015. **30**(8): p. 1105-1111.

[30] Weight, C.J., et al. *Physical activity, quality of life, and burnout among physician trainees: the effect of a team-based, incentivized exercise program.* in *Mayo Clinic Proceedings*. 2013. Elsevier.

[31] Ensor, K., M. Swaroop, and L. Tatebe, *Dealing with disruptive team members: Correcting" bad behaviors" while avoiding disruptions*, in *Fundamentals of Leadership for Healthcare Professionals*. 2018, Nova Science Publishers, Inc. p. 183-199.

[32] Tatebe, L. and M. Swaroop, *Disruptive physicians: How behavior can undermine patient safety.* Vignettes in Patient Safety, 2018. **2**: p. 273.

[33] Edmondson, A.C., *The kinds of teams health care needs.* Harv Bus Rev, 2015. **93**(12): p. 2-5.

[34] Edmondson, A.C., *The fearless organization: Creating psychological safety in the workplace for learning, innovation, and growth*. 2018: John Wiley & Sons.

[35] Papadimos, T.J., et al., *The importance of emotional intelligence to leadership in an academic health center.* International Journal of Academic Medicine, 2016. **2**(1): p. 57.

[36] Marcks, V., K. Hayes, and S.P. Stawicki, *Operating room trauma simulation: The St. Luke's University Health Network experience.* International Journal of Critical Illness and Injury Science, 2020. **10**(1): p. 4.

[37] Gale, J., S.P. Stawicki, and M. Swaroop, *Patient-Centered Transformation: Case Clinical Examples.* Fundamentals of Patient Safety in Medicine and Surgery, 2015: p. 142.

[38] Papadimos, T.J., E. Gafford, and S.P. Stawicki, *Empowering Engagement, Patients and Families: Candor, and Disclosure.* Fundamentals of Patient Safety in Medicine and Surgery, 2015: p. 205.

[39] Gillenwater, T. and L.M. King, *Lessons Healthcare Learned Systems from Best-Performing.* Fundamentals of Patient Safety in Medicine and Surgery, 2015: p. 275.

[40] Heerwagen, J.H., et al., *Collaborative knowledge work environments.* Building research & information, 2004. **32**(6): p. 510-528.

[41] Mintzberg, H., et al., *Some surprising things about collaboration-knowing how people connect makes it work better.* Organizational dynamics, 1996. **25**(1): p. 60-72.

[42] Grigsby, R., *Committee, task force, team: what's the difference? Why does it matter?* Academic Physician & Scientist, 2008: p. 4-5.

[43] Roach, D. *What Is The Difference Between a Committee and a Team*. 2020 [November 30, 2020]; Available from: https://likeateam.com/what-is-the-difference-between-a-committee-and-a-team/.

[44] Kaur, P. and J.C. Stoltzfuz, *All about governing stuctures and committees: Collective decision making in healthcare*, in *Fundamentals of Leadership for Healthcare Professionals*, S.P. Stawicki and M.S. Firstenberg, Editors. 2018, Nova Science Publishers: Hauppauge, NY. p. 241-260.

[45] Katzenbach, J.R. and D.K. Smith, *The wisdom of teams: Creating the high-performance organization*. 2015: Harvard Business Review Press.

[46] Sah, R.K. and J.E. Stiglitz, *Committees, hierarchies and polyarchies.* The Economic Journal, 1988. **98**(391): p. 451-470.

[47] Gerling, K., et al., *Information acquisition and decision making in committees: A survey.* European Journal of Political Economy, 2005. **21**(3): p. 563-597.

[48] Gibson, L.H. and P. Komlos-Hrobsky, *The Task Force as a Teaching Mechanism.* Clearinghouse Rev., 1984. **18**: p. 203.

[49] Falk, S., *Making citizen task forces work.* Public Management, 1993. **75**: p. 15-15.

[50] Neck, C.P. and C.C. Manz, *From groupthink to teamthink: Toward the creation of constructive thought patterns in self-managing work teams.* Human relations, 1994. **47**(8): p. 929-952.

[51] Janis, I.L., *Groupthink.* Psychology today, 1971. **5**(6): p. 43-46.

[52] Brookfield, S.D., *Teaching for critical thinking: Tools and techniques to help students question their assumptions*. 2011: John Wiley & Sons.

[53] Bowditch, J.L., A.F. Buono, and M.M. Stewart, *A primer on organizational behavior*. 2007: John Wiley & Sons.

[54] Foley, M., *Political leadership: Themes, contexts, and critiques*. 2013: Oxford University Press.

[55] Stawicki, S.P., N. Martins, and M.S. Firstenberg, *Leadership: What it is and what it isn't*, in *Fundamentals of Leadership for Healthcare Professionals - Volume 1*, S.P. Stawicki and M.S. Firstenberg, Editors. 2018, Nova Science Publishers: Hauppauge, NY.

[56] Tang, D., et al., *Headership in healthcare: From theory to practical application*, in *Fundamentals of Leadership for Healthcare Professionals*, S.P. Stawicki, M.S. Firstenberg, and T.J. Papadimos, Editors. 2019, Nova Science Publishers: Hauppauge, NY.

[57] Hargie, O., *Skilled interpersonal communication: Research, theory and practice*. 2010: Routledge.

[58] Hackman, J.R., *Collaborative intelligence: Using teams to solve hard problems*. 2011: Berrett-Koehler Publishers.

[59] Petrovich, M.V., *The Improvement Hierarchy.* Retrieved July, 2006. **5**.

[60] Lehman, P. *St. Luke's honors patients, first responders at 'Night of Heroes' event*. 2019 [December 12, 2020]; Available from: https://www.mcall.com/news/breaking/mc-nws-st-lukes-hospital-night-of-heroes-20190922-wg3xgru5i5h6zaqimfohimud4m-story.html.

[61] Stawicki, S.P., et al., *Retained surgical items: a problem yet to be solved.* Journal of the American College of Surgeons, 2013. **216**(1): p. 15-22.

[62] Moffatt-Bruce, S.D., et al., *Risk factors for retained surgical items: a meta-analysis and proposed risk stratification system.* journal of surgical research, 2014. **190**(2): p. 429-436.

[63] Stawicki, S.P., et al., *Natural history of retained surgical items supports the need for team training, early recognition, and prompt retrieval.* The American Journal of Surgery, 2014. **208**(1): p. 65-72.

[64] Wu, L., D. Wang, and J.A. Evans, *Large teams develop and small teams disrupt science and technology.* Nature, 2019. **566**(7744): p. 378-382.

[65] Kaba, A., et al., *Are we at risk of groupthink in our approach to teamwork interventions in health care?* Medical education, 2016. **50**(4): p. 400-408.

[66] Mao, A.T. and A.W. Woolley, *Teamwork in health care: maximizing collective intelligence via inclusive collaboration and open communication.* AMA journal of ethics, 2016. **18**(9): p. 933-940.

Chapter 2

The Impact of the Multidisciplinary Team on the Management of Prosthetic Joint Infection in Trauma and Orthopaedic Surgery

Nemandra A. Sandiford and Konrad Wronka

Abstract

Periprosthetic Joint Infection (PJI) is a devastating complication of the Total Joint Arthroplasty (TJA). It presents a great challenge for the clinician to diagnose and manage it appropriately, with significant morbidity for the patients and cost for health care providers. The purpose of this study is to review and examine the role of multi-disciplinary team (MDT) approach in diagnosis and management of prosthetic joint infection (PJI) and how this approach can influence outcomes. All published literature examining the role of multidisciplinary care in the management of PJI and the influence of this approach to the management and outcomes of patients with this diagnosis were included. Studies published in languages other than English were excluded. There is a paucity of data on the influence of multidisciplinary care on outcomes of the management of PJI. Evidence suggests that the MDT has important role in ensuring all factors in the management of this complex group are considered and best possible care is delivered. Multicentre randomised clinical trials are required to assess the influence of MDT'S on outcome as well as important questions around the structuring of these teams.

Keywords: prosthetic joint infection

1. Introduction and background

Prosthetic joint infection (PJI) affects about 1–3% of patients undergoing total joint arthroplasty [1]. In some units the infection rate is reported to be as high as 5% [2]. It is one of the most devastating complications and poses significant challenges for the patient, health care providers and the treating institution. The financial cost of treating a single case of PJI can be as high as £100,000 [2]. Costs for patients are even higher, with long hospital stay, multiple operations, associated pain and suffering, reduced life quality as well as risks associated with surgical morbidity and mortality. Diagnosis and management of PJI remains controversial and complex. There is no universal definition of the PJI. The definition

IntechOpen

of PJI proposed by the International Consensus Meeting on Periprosthetic Joint Infection is the most universally accepted one [3]. Other definitions also exist. George et al. [4] acknowledged 7 definitions produced by various consensus meetings. This illustrates that PJI remains a debatable and controversial topic and diagnosis is not straight forward. There is no one single test that can adequately diagnose PJI. Up to 10% of cases undergoing revision for aseptic loosening are later found to have prosthetic joint infection [5]. PJI can present in variety of ways and at varying phases from the time primary arthroplasty implantation. Tsukayama et al. proposed a classification system that divided PJI into four categories [6].

It can be challenging for an individual surgeon to make an accurate diagnosis when faced with a patient with a painful arthroplasty. One way of addressing this has been to manage this complex group of patients with a multidisciplinary team. Failure to make a timely and accurate diagnosis can significantly compromise therapeutic options and have a negative impact on the result of surgical treatment [7]. Furthermore, if PJI is not recognised, it may lead to systemic symptoms such as bacteraemia and septicaemia.

PJI can be challenging to treat, and patients may need a number of major surgical procedures, coupled with antimicrobial treatment for several weeks to eradicate the infection [8]. Treatment of PJI of the knee may be associated with a long period of disability with possible immobilisation of the knee. This may lead to a poor functional outcome. Recurrence of the infection is high and reported between 8% and 70% [9] and complications associated with surgery are common. Furthermore, PJI is associated with significant mortality. Berend et al. [10] reported that 11% patients treated for PJI with a 2 stage regime died between the first and second stages of surgical treatment. Zmistowski et al. [3] found that the 5-year survivorship of patients with PJI is worse than for some common cancers including breast cancer or testicular cancer. For this reason PJI must be managed expeditiously, providing patients with all available expertise to achieve the optimum outcome. Added to this is the psychological burden associated with the issues described and its impact on post operative function [11]. This combination of the knowledge that there has been a complication or suboptimal outcome, multiple surgical procedures, prolonged hospital stay, prolonged disability and associated medical comorbidities as well as social isolation and pain illustrates multiple issues which can be associated with patients presenting with PJI and the multiple facets which require management in a synchronised manner. These factors have been acknowledged in other aspects of orthopaedic surgery and it is acknowledged that optimal outcomes result from a multidisciplinary approach to management [12, 13].

2. Treatment options for PJI

Debridement, Antibiotics and Implant Retention (DAIR): When infection is diagnosed early, open debridement and exchange of modular prosthetic components followed by prolonged antibiotic therapy may lead to satisfactory results. Retention of the implant leads to superior functional results in cases where the infection is eradicated [14].

Single stage revision: Exchange off all components of the arthroplasty (both fixed and modular) is coupled with radical debridement of the joint and antibiotic treatment. Removal of all implants and reconstruction with new definitive prostheses. Single stage revision is usually performed in selected patients. The ideal patient is a well host, with a healthy soft tissue envelope, absence of a draining sinus and a known sensitive microbe are commonly accepted prerequisites [15].

Two stage revision: Removal of all implants during one surgical procedure is performed. The joint is excised with or without placement of a temporary spacer. Antibiotics are delivered locally (with cement or other delivery modes) and systemically. Following a prolonged period of antibiotic treatment (6 weeks or more), when infection is deemed to be eradicated, re-implantation (the second stage) is performed. During the second stage procedure further debridement takes place. The spacer is removed and the joint is reconstructed. The success rate is greater than of single stage revision procedure [10, 14]. The significant downside of this approach relates to the time between the 2 stages of the revision. During this time the patients' mobility is poor, joint function is very limited, and the patient is often required to stay in health care facility. The risk of complications (renal failure, *Clostridium difficile* diarrhoea) and mortality are significant. The patient also undergoes two separate major surgical procedures.

Excision arthroplasty: This involves removal of all the implants and excision of the joint followed by a course of antibiotics. The function of the joint is severely compromised, and the patient suffers significant disability. This salvage mode of treatment is reserved for the most complex infections in compromised hosts, with severe bone loss, presence of poly-microbial infection and an unhealthy soft tissue envelope exist [16].

Amputation: When the infection is not manageable or becomes a threat to the patient's life this might be the only option.

Prolonged suppressive antibiotic therapy (PSAT): In the presence of draining sinus and well-functioning joint, or when the host suffers from serious comorbidities that could preclude surgical intervention, antibiotic suppression may lead to satisfactory results. The infection cannot be eradicated, but it does not manifest itself systematically and symptoms related to the affected joint may be manageable for the patient. The senior author has previously reported found that infection control could be achieved in selected cases of PJI using this approach [17]. The patients' comorbidities and fitness for major surgery as well as psychological condition of the individual are also of incredible importance [18].

The physical, but also psychological needs of patients should be addressed. PJI may be emotionally difficult to cope with and lead to sequalae such as depression and anxiety [19]. Many patients struggle with the impact that the treatment of PJI has on their personal and family lives'. Patients' depression may require treatment and support during the treatment as well as during the recovery phases [20].

3. The role of the MDT

Ideally personnel should be present in the same location in order to provide a seamless, clinically and cost-efficient service to patients with PJI. They should be involved in all stages of the management pathways including, diagnosis, treatment (both surgical and non-surgical) and long term follow up. The multidisciplinary approach has made a significant difference in care of oncology patients. Time to diagnosis and clinical outcomes have all been shown to improve when the MDT functions well well [21, 22]. There is no published evidence to the authors' knowledge on the management of PJI with this approach however the principles of diagnosis and factors influencing management and outcomes of patients with PJI are similar. It seems intuitive therefore that a similar approach to treatment might produce similar outcomes.

4. What comprises a multidisciplinary team?

Most published studies examining the benefits of MDT's have focused on clinical results [22]. There is a relative paucity of data on the components of the MDT. An important principle of care delivery in this setting is consideration of the wholistic needs of the patient and including appropriate specialists to address these issues. In the context of PJI the following team members are required:

Orthopaedic Surgeon- The surgeon coordinates and orchestrates the care of the patient. They need to establish the diagnosis, identify the individuals required to care for the patient and coordinate meetings. They are required to have the necessary skillset and to carry out the surgical treatment required. A minimum requirement would be fellowship training in revision arthroplasty surgery.

Microbiologist- A microbiologist is vital to the multidisciplinary team. With their expertise and specialist knowledge of microbial metabolism specific diagnostic requirements, mechanism of antibiotic function and interactions and the requirements for monitoring of these issues, their importance is non controversial. The role of musculoskeletal microbiology is rapidly evolving with developments in diagnosis such as 16 s polymerase chain reaction (16 s PCR) testing. This speciality has made significant contributions to the practical management of patients with PJI such as the OVIVA (Oral versus Intravenous Antibiotics for Bone and Joint Infection) trial [23]. A dedicated microbiology clinic also provides another medium for follow up and support of this complex group of patients.

Musculoskeletal Radiologist- Radiologists are central in the decision making process. This stage often requires judgement based on a variety of imaging modalities. An experienced radiologist is invaluable in advising on the optimal imaging modality and interpreting subtle signs on imaging. In the experience of the authors this is one of the most useful and educational parts of the MDT meeting.

Nutritionist- Nutritionists contribute significantly to pre and post operative optimisation of the patient. Malnutrition and vitamin D deficiency have been shown to positively correlate with PJI [24]. Low serum albumin level and low lymphocyte count are at increased risk of infection, wound dehiscence and medical complications [25–27]. Cross et al. [26] postulated that normalisation of the serum albumin level and tight glucose control may lead to better outcomes in orthopaedic surgery. Management of these factors has an important role in reducing the risk of reinfection following revision surgery.

Physiotherapist- The ultimate aim of revision surgery is restoration of a pain free, mobile with restoration of function and activity. Pre and post operative physiotherapy is vital to achieving these aims. Physical therapy has been shown to improve soft-tissue tension, joint range of motion, and muscle strength and can reduce pain and stiffness [28, 29].

Clinical Nursing Specialist (CNS)- The role of a dedicated nurse specialist care cannot be understated. Walker [30] acknowledged the vital role which nurses play in the management of patients undergoing joint replacement surgery. The multifaceted role of a CNS has also been described by Pertino et al. [31]. The nurse specialist has several key clinical and organisational roles including being the point of contact for referrals, organising investigations, coordinating care between multiple specialities when these are involved and being a point of contact for patients.

5. Examples of multidisciplinary teams

At the authors' institution, there is an established referral network for complex cases including those presenting with PJI. Clinicians from the region can refer any patient who needs complex arthroplasty assessment and treatment, including those with PJI to a centralised hub. There is a standardised referral proforma and MDT coordinator who promptly responds to all referrals. There is a weekly MDT attended by complex arthroplasty surgeons, a CNS and radiologists with an interest in musculoskeletal medicine. Cases are discussed and either advice is provided or a decision on transfer of the patient to the Hub Hospital is organised. In complex cases when surgery is required, surgical planning is performed and details such as surgical approach, instruments and required implants are all discussed. Each week between 10 to 20 cases are discussed. Advice of plastic surgeons, vascular surgeons and microbiologists is available on request. There is also a monthly MDT meeting attended by the same team of complex arthroplasty surgeons as well as microbiologists with an interest in bone and joint infection and outpatient antibiotic treatment (OPAT) team. All cases undergoing treatment for infection are discussed, plans for surgical and non-surgical treatment are established and progress of treated patients is discussed. This ensures that most appropriate treatment plan is made for each individual.

The East Midlands Specialist Orthopaedic Network (EMSON) (Nottingham, UK) was established and its success has been reported [32]. All referrals are received by email by the MDT coordinator. The meetings are conducted using secure videolink, with complex arthroplasty surgeons from Nottingham University Hospital and microbiologists attending while consultants from neighbouring hospitals dial in to discuss challenging cases. During first 6 months 166 cases were discussed, 43% of which the initial plan was amended as the result of the discussion. In several cases, there was a significant alteration to the treatment plan. Referring surgeons are also encouraged to come to tertiary centre with the potential for joint consultant operating. This improves the experience of all clinicians involved.

6. Why should we adopt a Multidisciplinary approach

The potential benefits of care delivered via a MDT approach can be experienced on a variety of levels:

The Unit level- The centre which provides this level of care will likely benefit from an increased volume of patients and referrals. This will the increase the experience gained by clinicians in dealing with his condition.

The clinician level- Individual clinicians will have improved exposure to a larger number of cases. This has the potential to improve technical proficiency. Clinicians will also be motivated to receive further training and broaden their knowledge in field of PJI. This will also improve their knowledge and level of expertise by participating in MDT discussions.

The patient level- Patients are more likely to receive coordinated, individual care by specialists with greatest level of expertise in the field of PJI.

7. Challenges to the establishment of a multidisciplinary team

The treatment of PJI is labour and resource intensive. Patients often stay on the ward for extended periods and face a higher risk of surgical and medical complications that non-infected cases. It is likely that the number of referrals and number of treated patients will increase over time which increases this burden [32].

Vaneghan et al. have shown that the cost of surgical treatment is significantly higher than septic revisions [33]. There is a potential risk of rapid depletion of financial resources. Renumeration strategies need to be established prior to starting this type of service [18, 33].

The logistics and practical aspects of establishing a MDT requires careful attention to detail. An understanding of what is required on a practical level is important. Meetings of large numbers of specialists takes these services from other departments. To the authors' knowledge there has been no definition of the optimal constituents a MDT or of the minimal number of specialists required or whether the teams involved in diagnostic and therapeutic parts of the patient journey should be different.

Job planning for all the members of the team should be coordinated to allow all members to meet or dial in to discuss cases. Surgeons, radiologists, microbiologists and other health care professionals involved in PJI management need to find time during their busy weekly schedule for MDT to work. Furthermore, when transfer of the patient is necessary to the specialist centre, logistical arrangements need to be in place to avoid delays.

Another unexplored aspect of delivering care in this way is the issue of responsibility and autonomy. The MDT moves away from the heirarchical system in which decisions are made by one senior individual towards one where there is shared decision making. This raises the subject of accountability. When a decision is taken by a group, who is responsible and who, if anyone, is accountable when things go wrong? For the same reason there can be a perceived risk to the autonomy of the referring surgeon. These issues have not been addressed.

In conclusion the management of PJI is complex and multifactorial. Multidisciplinary management has resulted in improved clinical results in similar settings setting such as tumour surgery however establishment of multidisciplinary care presents significant challenges to the treating institution.

Author details

Nemandra A. Sandiford[1]* and Konrad Wronka[2]

1 Trauma and Orthopaedic Surgery, Southland Teaching Hospital, Invercargill, New Zealand

2 Trauma and Orthopaedics, Prince Philip Hospital, Llanelli, GBR

*Address all correspondence to: nemsandiford@gmail.com

IntechOpen

© 2020 The Author(s). Licensee IntechOpen. This chapter is distributed under the terms of the Creative Commons Attribution License (http://creativecommons.org/licenses/by/3.0), which permits unrestricted use, distribution, and reproduction in any medium, provided the original work is properly cited. CC BY

References

[1] https: //www.hqip.org.uk/wp-content/uploads/2018/11/NJR-15th-Annual-Report-2018.pdf (last accessed 5-05-2020)

[2] Blom A, Brown J, Taylor AH et al. Infection after total knee arthroplasty. J Bone Joint Surg Br. 2004;86(5):688-91.

[3] Briggs T. W. (2015). A national review of adult elective orthopaedic services in England. Getting it right first time. Retrieved from http://www.gettingitrightfirsttime.com/downloads/GIRFT-National-Report.pdf [last accessed 23 June 2016].

[4] Parvizi J,Gehrke T, Chen A. Proceedings of the International Consensus on Periprosthetic Joint Infection. Bone Joint J 2013;95-B:1450-2.

[5] Tansey R, Mirza Y, Sukeik M et al. Definition of Periprosthetic Hip and Knee Joint Infections and the Economic Burden. Open Orthop J. 2016;10:662-668.

[6] Tsukayama DT, Goldberg VM, Kyle R. Diagnosis and management of infection after total knee arthroplasty. J Bone Joint Surg Am. 2003;85-A Suppl 1:S75-80.

[7] Saleh A, Guirguis A, Klika A et al. Unexpected Positive Intraoperative Cultures in Aseptic Revision Arthroplasty The Journal of Arthroplasty . 2014; 29:2181-2186.

[8] Tande AJ, Patel R. Prosthetic joint infection. Clin Microbiol Rev. 2014;27(2):302-45.

[9] M. Marín, J. M. Garcia-Lechuz, P. Alonso et al. Role of Universal 16S rRNA Gene PCR and Sequencing in Diagnosis of Prosthetic Joint Infection. Journal of Clinical Microbiology 2012; 50 (3) 583-589.

[10] Yi PH, Cross MB, Moric M et al. The 2013 Frank Stinchfield Award: Diagnosis of infection in the early postoperative period after total hip arthroplasty. Clin Orthop Relat Res. 2014;472(2):424-429.

[11] Deirmengian C, Kardos K, Kilmartin P et al. Diagnosing periprosthetic joint infection: has the era of the biomarker arrived?. Clin Orthop Relat Res. 2014;472(11):3254-3262.

[12] Moore AJ, Whitehouse MR, Gooberman-Hill R et al. A UK national survey of care pathways and support offered to patients receiving revision surgery for prosthetic joint infection in the highest volume NHS orthopaedic centres. Musculoskeletal Care. 2017;15(4):379-385.

[13] Kunutsor SK, Whitehouse MR, Lenguerrand E et al. Re-Infection Outcomes Following One- And Two-Stage Surgical Revision of Infected Knee Prosthesis: A Systematic Review and Meta-Analysis. PLoS One. 2016;11:11(3).

[14] Berend KR, Lombardi AV Jr, Morris MJ et al. Two-stage treatment of hip periprosthetic joint infection is associated with a high rate of infection control but high mortality. Clin Orthop Relat Res. 2013;471(2):510-8.

[15] Zmistowski B, Karam JA, Durinka JB et al. Periprosthetic joint infection increases the risk of one-year mortality. J Bone Joint Surg Am. 2013;95(24):2177-84.

[16] Boettner F, Cross MB, Nam D et al. Functional and emotional results differ after aseptic vs septic revision hip arthroplasty. HSS J 2011;7(3):235-238.

[17] Vaishya R, Agarwal AK, Rawat SK et al. Is Single-stage Revision Safe Following Infected Total Knee

Arthroplasty? A Critical Review. Cureus. 2017;9(8):e1629.

[18] Shanmugasundaram S, Ricciardi BF, Briggs TW et al. Evaluation and Management of Periprosthetic Joint Infection-an International, Multicenter Study. HSS J. 2014;10(1):36-44.

[19] https://icmphilly.com/questions/does-arthroscopic-surgery-have-any-role-in-the-treatment-of-acute-or-chronic-periprosthetic-joint-infection-pji-of-the-knee-or-the-hip/ (Last accessed 22/05/2020)

[20] Hamblen DL. Diagnosis of infection and the role of permanent excision arthroplasty. Orthop Clin North Am. 1993;24(4):743-9.

[21] Prendki V, Zeller V, Passeron D et al. Outcome of patients over 80 years of age on prolonged suppressive antibiotic therapy for at least 6 months for prosthetic joint infection. Int J Infect Dis. 2014;29:184-9.

[22] Parvizi J, Zmistowski B, Adeli B. Periprosthetic joint infection: treatment options. Orthopedics. 2010;33(9):659.

[23] Sandiford NA, Hutt JR, Kendoff DO et al. Prolonged suppressive antibiotic therapy is successful in the management of prosthetic joint infection. Eur J Orthop Surg Traumatol. 2020;30(2):313-321.

[24] Moore A J, Blom AW, Whitehouse MR et al. Deep prosthetic joint infection: a qualitative study of the impact on patients and their experiences of revision surgery. BMJ Open; 5(12): e009495.

[25] Birchall M, Bailey D, King P. South West Cancer Intelligence Service Head and Neck Tumour Panel: Effect of process standards on survival of patients with head and neck cancer in the south and west of England. Br J Cancer 2004;91(8):1477-1481.

[26] Croke JM, El-Sayed S: Multidisciplinary management of cancer patients: Chasing a shadow or real value? An overview of the literature. Curr Oncol 2012;19(4): e232-e238.

[27] Scarborough M, Li HK, Rombach I, et al. Oral versus intravenous antibiotics for bone and joint infections: the OVIVA non-inferiority RCT. *Health Technol Assess*. 2019;23(38):1-92.

[28] Namba RS, Inacio MC, Paxton EW. Risk factors associated with deep surgical site infections after primary total knee arthroplasty: an analysis of 56,216 knees. J. Bone Joint Surg. Am. 95:775-782. 10.2106/JBJS.L.00211.

[29] Bohl DD, Shen MR, Kayupov E et al. Hypoalbuminemia Independently Predicts Surgical Site Infection, Pneumonia, Length of Stay, and Readmission After Total Joint Arthroplasty. J Arthroplasty. 2016 Jan;31(1):15-21.

[30] Cross MB, Yi PH, Thomas CF et al. Evaluation of malnutrition in orthopaedic surgery. J Am Acad Orthop Surg. 2014 Mar;22(3):193-9.

[31] Snow R, Granata J, Ruhil AV et al. Associations between preoperative physical therapy and post-acute care utilization patterns and cost in total joint replacement. J Bone Joint Surg Am. 2014 Oct 1;96(19):e165.

[32] Walker J. Care of patients undergoing joint replacement. Nurs Older People.2012 Feb;24(1):14-20.

[33] Bloch B, Raglan M, Manktelow, A et al. The East Midlands Specialist Orthopaedic Network: the future of revision arthroplasty?. The Bulletin of the Royal College of Surgeons of England. 99. 66-70. 10.1308/rcsbull.2017.66.

Chapter 3

Teamwork in Healthcare Management

Mercè Mach, António C.M. Abrantes and Ceferí Soler

Abstract

Groups are pervasive in healthcare institutions and take on a variety of shapes. This paper uses a typology that allows us to understand the distinctive characteristics of team operations, based on interdependence and interactive dimensions. It looks at factors that influence team effectiveness in organizational settings. We review different frameworks that shed light in explaining the conditions that lead to group effectiveness. From the classical input-process-output (IPO) model to the input-mediator-output-input (IMOI) model of team effectiveness; the taxonomy of team process and emergent estates, as well as the teams understood as complex adaptive systems and also studied from the multiteam system perspective. We also report the need for more robust research designs to contribute to the field's further advancement. There is consensus among scholars demanding further conceptual frameworks, as well as powerful research designs that capture process-oriented theory and research on team effectiveness. Some future directions and recommendations are suggested.

Keywords: teamwork, interaction, interdependence, effectiveness

1. Introduction

In recent decades, organizations have increasingly turned to using teams and made them a part of day-to-day routines [1, 2], and all for a variety of reasons, such as the ability to respond to emergencies, engage in continuous quality improvement efforts, and manage work projects through multidisciplinary teams. In the particular case of healthcare organizations, teamwork is essential to provide effective care, and the lack of teamwork has been identified in the literature as a key vulnerability in terms of service quality [3, 4]. In this chapter we propose revisiting the conditions that promote effective teamwork. We will first examine team work typology, using interaction and interdependence as the key dimensions characterizing and describing teams. We will then focus on teamwork effectiveness and review a few of the more influential frameworks that have driven research dedicated to teams. Finally, we will conclude with some directions for future teamwork research. But, first, we should briefly discuss what a team and teamwork are.

Kozlowski and Ilgen [5] provide a rather thorough definition of teams, describing them as "two or more individuals who socially interact (face-to-face or, increasingly, virtually); possess one or more common goals; are brought together to perform organizationally relevant tasks; exhibit interdependencies with respect to workflow, goals, and outcomes; have different roles and responsibilities; and are together embedded in an encompassing organizational system, with boundaries and linkages to the broader system context and task environment" (p. 79) [5]. Although exhaustive, this approach defines teams in a somewhat mechanistic way in terms of their design, with an external focus. This view has been countered with a different perspective which sees teams as more dynamic and as self-constructed entities. This led Humprey and Amy [6] to define teams as "assemblies of interdependent relations and activities organizing shifting sets or subsets of participants embedded in and relevant to wider resource and institutional environments" (p. 450) [6].

On the other hand, teamwork is a process that emerges from the interactions established among team members [7] and it can be defined as "a set of interrelated thoughts, actions, and feelings of each team member that are needed to function as a team and that combine to facilitate coordinated, adaptive performance and task objectives resulting in value-added outcomes" (p. 562) [8]. Teamwork reflects the minute-by-minute behaviours and interactions that take place between team members work when executing a task [9]. As proposed by Salas et al. [9], teamwork is guided by a number of fundamental principles: it is characterized by a set of behaviours, cognitions and attitudes that should be flexible and adaptive; team members should monitor each other and feel safe to provide feedback and comfortable when receiving it; team members should also be willing and capable of providing support to other team members in their operations and activities; teamwork involves clear, precise, and concise communication; team members must be able to coordinate interdependently to take collective action; teamwork requires leadership that provides direction, planning, distribution, and activity coordination; and, finally, teamwork is subject to external influences as well as to the requirements of the task itself.

2. Typology of formal groups

As in all organizations, groups are pervasive in healthcare institutions and take on a variety of shapes, ranging from different units or working groups that are permanent in nature to "ad hoc" groups (committees, meetings, etc.) which are eminently temporary. In order to manage this variety of groups, establishing a typology will allow us to understand the distinctive characteristics of their operations. In addition to varying relative to the purposes they serve, formal groups (permanent or temporary) also diverge according to the basic characteristics of how they operate. The way they function is determined by two basic dimensions: team interaction and interdependence. Team interaction relates to how team members "behav[e] together, in some recognized relation to one another" (p. 12) [10], for the purpose of performing a task. Team interdependence is the extent to which team members cooperate, depend on each other, and work interactively to complete team tasks [11]. Although related, the two concepts are independent in the sense that, although teams with high degrees of interdependence also have high degrees of interaction, the same does not always happen in the opposite sense. That is, teams with a high degree of interaction do not necessarily have a high degree of interdependence, since team members may interact but not depend on each other.

2.1 Team interaction

Team interaction is central to teamwork and represents complex, temporal phenomena with multilevel manifestations [12]. It is complex because it involves a web of behavioural connections between team members; it is temporal because the very execution of team tasks has a temporal dimension unfolding over time at a specific rhythm and pace; and it manifests at several levels because it is nested in individual and collective behaviours. Team interaction is thus subject to influences from elements related to individuals, from elements within the team itself, and from relational factors. Individual factors can include, for example, team members' attitudes towards work and the team. Collaborative attitudes will promote better interactions than competitive ones. Regarding team factors, for example, Lehmann-Willenbrock and Allen [13] observed that humour considered at the team level has a positive influence on the incidence of interactions within the team. From a relational point of view, differences in status and power within the team also influence the level of interaction, with that interaction increasing the smaller the differences in status and power. The team's interaction level also has significant and positive outcomes for teams. One such consequence is the development of similar team mental models, which can be defined as a common understanding among team members about key elements in the relevant team environment [14]. The similarity of team mental models has positive effects on several dimensions such as team performance [15] and adaptive capacity [16].

2.2 Team interdependence

Although team interdependence can be considered a single general factor, it can also be seen in three distinct dimensions: task, goal, and outcome interdependence [17]. *Task interdependence* concerns the degree of task-induced interactions between members; *goal interdependence* refers to the relationships between members arising from the type of goal (whether individual or team, for example) that drives members' performance and efforts; *outcome interdependence* refers to interdependent feedback and rewards as they relate to individual or collective performance. These types of interdependence have different consequences on team performance. For example, in a meta-analysis, Courtright et al. [18] concluded that task and outcome interdependence affect performance via different mechanisms. Task interdependence is primarily associated with team performance through its effects on team functioning in relation to the task, such as through actions or transition processes or through team-efficacy. Contrarily, outcome interdependence is mainly associated with team performance through its effects on team functioning in relation to relational aspects, such as interpersonal processes or cohesion. However, although distinct, these three types of interdependence are highly related. As Gully et al. [17] argue, when team members are performing a highly interdependent task, they tend to have interdependent goals and outcomes.

In particular, task interdependence has been widely studied [19, 20] for its implications on the way teams operate and perform. For example, to determine how to assign outcomes to individual group members, the types of tasks the team performs have to be taken into account. Thompson's [21] group task model (**Figure 1**) can help to assess the extent to which the work performed by one member affects what other group members do, as well as identifying the most effective way to distribute outcomes and/or rewards. In essence, this model reveals the form that task interdependence can take.

In the *pooled interdependence* type of task, members only depend on each other because they belong to the same organization or department. Each member of the group makes a separate and independent contribution to overall team performance. They may compete for resources but, generally, they operate relatively independently [21]. There is little interaction among members and there are few potentially dysfunctional consequences. This pooled interdependence generates additive outputs. Classic examples include a group of sales representative in a pharmaceutical company or a group of physicians in a healthcare centre.

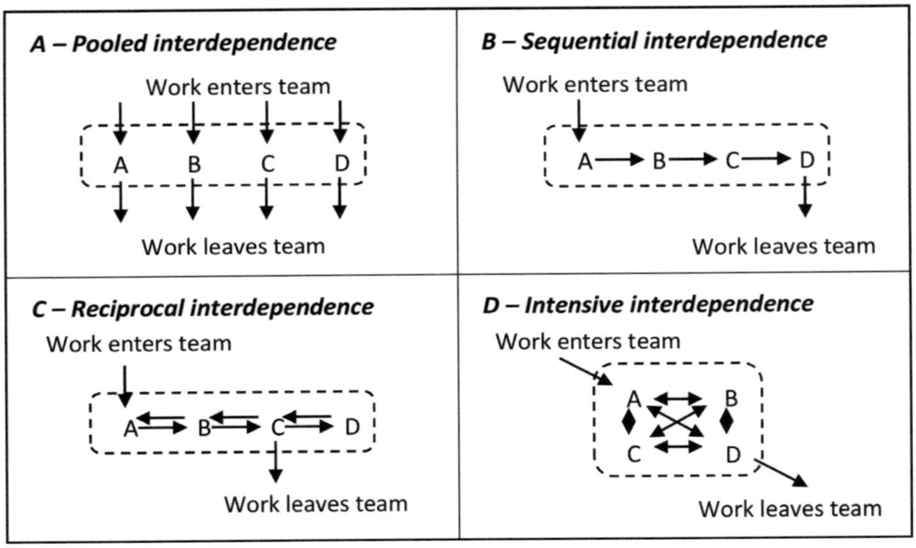

Figure 1.
Types of task interdependence (based on Thompson model of group task [21]).

Group tasks based on *sequential interdependence* require specific behaviours to be performed by the group's members in a predetermined order. The level of each member's performance, consequently, affects the performance of other members down the line. In this type of task, members' outputs are required for the following members to perform their duties. Problems arise if the first members do not perform their jobs effectively, potentially leading to the following members having to adopt defensive strategies. When group members' activities are sequentially interdependent, the performance level of the least capable or poorest-performing member of the group determines overall group performance [21]. Examples of sequential interdependence include any kind of assembly-line work, where the finished product is the result of all the group members' sequential inputs.

In tasks with *reciprocal interdependence*, the activities of all the work group's members are fully dependent on one another, so that each member's performance influences the performance of every other group member. Work groups performing tasks characterized by this reciprocal interdependence tend to experience considerable coordination problems due to unpredictable group relations and interactions. There is no set ordering of the group's activities when its tasks are organized reciprocally, unlike when tasks are organized in a sequential manner [21]. An example of reciprocal interdependence could be the protocols established for organ transplant surgery.

Intensive interdependence is one step ahead of reciprocal interdependence. This type of interdependence implies a fully connected communication network. Each group member's activities precede and are required for all the other group members' activities. Groups with this type of interdependence have the greatest potential for conflict, and they require the greatest number of effective communication mechanisms [21]. Examples of work groups whose tasks are intensively interdependent include operating room teams in hospitals, top management teams, emergency room teams, and R&D teams.

With increasing interdependence –pooled interdependence, sequential, reciprocal, and intensive–, the potential for conflict and dysfunctional behaviours can increase [22]. However, research provides strong evidence that the relationship between team efficacy (team perceptions regarding its ability to perform a specific task) and performance is stronger when that interdependence is high compared to when it is low [17].

2.3 Types of groups

Based on the two team interaction and interdependence dimensions, we can distinguish four types of organisational groups (**Figure 2**): Staff/Crew, Remote-controlled group, Coordinated group, and Team. In the *Staff/Crew* type of group there is proximity or social contact between the people who make up the group, although their tasks are not interdependent. This group's results are generally additive, that is, they correspond to the sum of the individual members' results. Contrarily, there is no interaction or interdependence among the members in a *Remote-controlled group*. The group is merely 'nominal' and exists for the purposes of the organization, but it does not act as a group in terms of the work conducted by its members. In the *Coordinated group* there is no direct contact between its members, although they may depend on each other to carry out their work. And the *Team* group is characterised by a high degree of interaction and interdependence among its members.

2.4 Nature of team tasks

There are numerous dimensions by which tasks can be classified. Above we saw a classification based on interdependence, but we can look at tasks from another perspective, for example, according to the team members' contributions. From this standpoint, tasks can be additive, conjunctive or disjunctive [23]. A task is *additive* when the group's success depends on the sum of the individual group members' performance. Additive tasks are divisible, and the group's performance is a function of the average competence of the individuals within it. For additive tasks, the group's potential performance increases with the size of the group. A typical example of an additive task is a relay race, in which the final result represents the sum of each member's performance. In general, more people putting in more effort will result in a better outcome. For example, a hospital's emergency room triage team performs an additive type of task when we consider the number of triaged patients as a measure of its performance. This number represents the sum of each triage team member's performance.

Conjunctive tasks are those requiring all group members to contribute to complete the product or output. The group task cannot be completed successfully

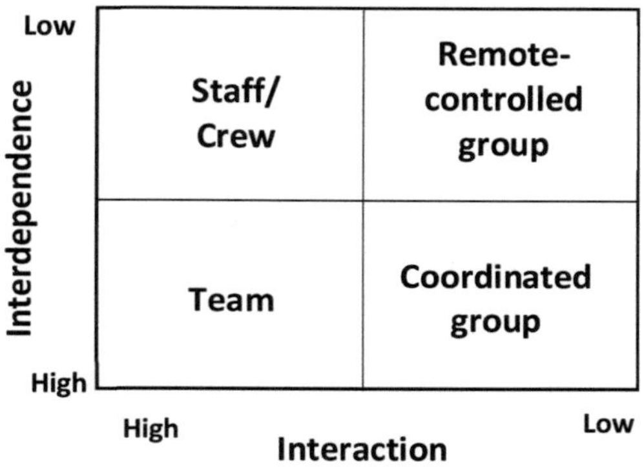

Figure 2.
Types of groups based on team interaction and interdependence dimensions.

until all the members have finalized their portion of the job. This means that the speed and quality of the group's performance are determined by the least skilled or inferior member, such as in an assembly-line which is limited by its weakest link. Both potential and actual performance of conjunctive tasks decreases as group size increases. An example of a conjunctive task could be a taskforce to develop a new protocol to resolve bottlenecks in a hospital emergency room, in which each group member has specific knowledge without which the task cannot be completed [24].

A *disjunctive task* is one in which the group's performance depends on the performance by the best member of the group, typically a task involving decision-making or problem-solving. One example is a research team looking for a single error in a complicated computer program. Disjunctive tasks require group members to define a single solution or make a decision or recommendation that will be adopted on behalf of the entire group. This means that the group's performance tends to be determined by the most skilled or logical-minded member. The potential performance of groups performing disjunctive tasks increases with group size. In the healthcare industry, an example of a disjunctive task is a weekly clinical case meeting in a hospital (or its online version). Disjunctive tasks predominate in the coordinated groups and teams seen above, although conjunctive tasks are also frequently performed by these types of groups [23].

In this section we have looked at some typologies of formal groups and discussed the interdependence of the teams' tasks and their members' interaction. In the next section we will review some of the most influential frameworks driving research on work teams.

3. Approaches to team dynamics

The last three decades have seen a significant increase in the number of articles published on teams or groups. A literature review of articles published in the *Journal of Applied Psychology* over the last century found that studies referring to groups or teams have more than quadrupled since the 1990s [25]. Numerous studies have been carried out to shed light on which specific set of characteristics and processes possibly lead to effective team outcomes [6]. Today, we know a lot about teams and their dynamics: we know what influences them, how to develop them, how to lead them and make them more cohesive; we also know that to be effective they have to be adaptable and flexible [26]. Teams are complex dynamic systems that develop over time as their members evolve and adapt to the different situational demands they continually face [5]. Therefore, they are strongly influenced by a wide range of factors that make teams different in a variety of ways, from their skills and level of virtuality to their culture and personality [26]. Let's look at some factors that influence team effectiveness.

3.1 Fundamental frameworks

Scholars have developed different frameworks to attempt to explain the conditions that lead to group effectiveness. The classic input-process-output (IPO) model of team effectiveness [27, 28] guided developments in team research for several decades. Within the IPO model, the inputs are the antecedents, that is, the conditions that exist prior to the group activity (e.g., organizational context, task characteristics, and team composition). The processes are the interactions among group members that mediate the relationship between the team's inputs and outputs (e.g., communication and coordination processes). Lastly, the outputs are the results, the consequences of group activity (e.g., productivity/performance, member satisfaction, and innovation). For example, the early IPO model proposed by McGrath [28] suggests that individual, group, and environmental-level factors are antecedents to group interaction processes with effects on performance outcomes such as quality, speed, number of errors, and other types of outcomes, such as member satisfaction or group cohesion.

The IPO model has been highly influential in research on teams and how members can combine their efforts and knowledge to complete a specific task. However, more recently, the model has been questioned as it has some limitations when considering the dynamic nature of teams [29, 30]. One criticism raised is that, despite involving team interactions, many researchers studying processes only assess these as static retrospective perceptions, ignoring how they emerge, their dynamics and evolution over time [29]. Furthermore, the IPO model does not take into account that all mediational factors are not necessarily processes but can also be emergent states [31] as we explore below. In addition, teamwork influences create a feedback loop in which reversal causal sequences are also possible, given that the results of a team's actions can also be an input for the following action, something not reflected in IPO models [31, 32]. To avoid some of these limitations, Ilgen, et al. [33] proposed the input-mediator-output-input (IMOI) model. In the latter, inputs are added at the end of the model to denote the system's cyclical nature, and processes are replaced by mediators to reflect a wider range of variables, namely processes and emergent states.

3.2 Team processes and emergent states

As seen above, not all team mediation mechanisms are processes; some are emergent states [31] . The difference between the two is fundamental, since processes imply interactions while emergent states do not. *Team processes* reflect the different types of activities and interactions that occur within a team and contribute to its end goals. They can be defined as "members' interdependent acts that convert inputs to outcomes through cognitive, verbal, and behavioral activities directed toward organizing task work to achieve collective goals" (p. 357) [31]. On the other hand, *emergent states* are an epiphenomenon (by-product) that results from the interaction between team members. Marks et al. [31] define them as "properties of the team that are typically dynamic in nature and vary as a function of team context, inputs, processes, and outcomes" (p. 357) [31]. Thus, when implementing processes, team members operate interdependently using the various resources at their disposal to achieve the team's objectives. For example, these resources may be their own competencies or the equipment they have available. As for emergent states, they are a product of the team's experiences and reflect its cognitive, motivational, and affective states. Although they are a product of interactions and, therefore, of processes, emergent states are also inputs to subsequent processes and outcomes.

This sequential notion in which a process or emergent state is both an output and an input of subsequent processes and emergent states leads us to the recurring phase model of team processes proposed by Marks et al. [31]. In their model, team performance episodes unfold over time, signalling specific periods in which action and transition phases occur. *Action phases* are periods of time in which teams are actively involved in executing a task, trying to achieve the proposed objectives. The teams' actions depend on their nature. For example, surgical teams perform operations; emergency medical teams treat acute patients without prior appointment; firefighting teams put out fires; and research teams collect and analyse data. *Transition phases* occur between the different action phases. In these transition phases, teams focus on evaluating the previous action phase and planning the next one. These are periods of reflection where actual and projected performance levels are compared and potential performance gaps are addressed. In each of these phases there is an IPO model, that is, a set of processes that have antecedents and that result in outputs for the next phase. For example, a given action phase's performance quality is the input for the next transition phase. Antecedents such as member diversity, task interdependence, and team size affect team processes that, in turn, have a strong impact on team effectiveness and performance.

Marks et al. [31] developed a taxonomy of team processes that considers practices that typically occur in transition phases, those that occur in action phases, and interpersonal processes that occur in both. In transition phases, team members conduct three types of processes: mission analysis, goal specification, and strategy formulation. *Mission analysis* processes refer to teams interpreting and evaluating their mission and identifying their main tasks, the operational context, and available resources; *goal specification* processes imply team members identifying and prioritising their goals and subgoals; and, lastly, *strategy formulation* processes include developing alternative courses of action to accomplish the mission, as well as defining contingency plans in case there is any change in the context. Typical processes in the action phase include progress, system and team monitoring as well as backup behaviours and coordination. *Progress monitoring* consists of overseeing the task and checking its progress; *system monitoring* implies tracking internal systems such as equipment or personnel and tracking external systems, for example, changes in the environment; *team monitoring and backup behaviours* refer to actions to help other team members perform their tasks (ranging from simple verbal feedback to replacing a colleague in performing a task); and, finally, *coordination* refers to orchestrating the sequence and synchronisation of interdependent actions. Coordination can be explicit, which implies that team members communicate with each other overtly, but it can also be implicit, consisting of the team's ability to act collectively, with members anticipating the needs of the task and other members and adjusting their behaviour accordingly, without the need to communicate overtly [34]. There are, however, other types of processes which may occur either in action or transition phases and which refer to processes that regulate interpersonal activities, that is, interpersonal processes. These comprise conflict management, motivation, and confidence building, as well as affect management. *Conflict management* can be both preventive, establishing the conditions to prevent, control, or guide conflict before it occurs, and reactive, which is a way of resolving conflicts when they do occur; *motivation and confidence building* consist of creating and maintaining a collective feeling of confidence, motivation, and cohesion, that is, creating emergent states that are positive for the mission; and *affect management* refers to regulating members' emotions when working.

Recently, Mathieu, Luciano et al. [35] have developed a team process survey tool that allows researchers to examine team processes more systematically (transition, action, and interpersonal processes). In its more extensive version, this tool includes 50 items, while its intermediate version has 30 and the reduced version only 10, one for each process. As recommended by authors [35], the use of the reduced 10-item version may be tempting, but it is not the most appropriate in all situations. The longer versions offer a more complete representation of the various dimensions. For example, Marks et al.'s taxonomy [31] includes several sub-processes that are not revealed in the 10-item version. When the aim is to get an in-depth view of the team's processes, the 30- and 50-item versions are more advisable. When only a quick look at how the team currently functions is desired or when this measure is included in a more extensive questionnaire along with other scales, using the 10-item version may be advantageous.

With regard to emergent states, an article by Grossman, Friedman and Kalra [36] summarises the emergent states emphasized the most in the literature, dividing them into affective and cognitive mechanisms. In *affective mechanisms* we find cohesion, confidence, and trust; *cognitive mechanisms* consist of team mental models and transactive memory systems. *Team cohesion* is one of the most studied emergent states in team literature and across a wide range of disciplines, from sports psychology [37, 38], to military psychology [39]. It is "a dynamic process which is reflected in the tendency for a group to stick together and remain united in the pursuit of its goals and objectives" (p. 124) [40]. In the particular case of teams operating in highly stressful or very task-oriented environments, such as healthcare, research has shown that team cohesion is crucial for team performance [41]. *Team confidence* includes team efficacy and team potency. These two constructs are similar but distinct. While team efficacy refers to the shared belief that the team can perform a certain task, team potency refers to the belief about the team's ability to be successful in different tasks and contexts. Both dimensions have a positive effect on team performance, especially team efficacy, particularly when tasks are highly interdependent [17]. *Team trust* refers to the team members' shared willingness to be vulnerable to other members' actions [42, 43]. Without trust, team members are unlikely to be able to work effectively with each other. These three mechanisms, though independent, have some interactions. For example, Mach et al. [38] observed that team trust has an effect on performance through team cohesion. In other words, the greater the team trust, the more cohesive teams are, which contributes positively to their performance.

As far as cognitive mechanisms are concerned, *team mental models* play a major role. These are shared representations of key elements concerning the task environment, whether related to the task, to the team itself or even to temporal aspects [14, 44]. As seen above, team mental models have a positive effect on several team outcomes, from performance to adaptation. Another cognitive mechanism is the *transactive memory system*, which refers to a shared system that combines each member's memory system with a shared understanding of what each member knows and for what kind of knowledge they are responsible, that is, who knows what [45, 46]. In addition, this emergent state contributes to teams' successful performance [45], as it allows lightening each team member's cognitive load and also expands the pool of expertise and knowledge available. Emergent processes and states interplay with mutual precedence relations as well as with interaction relations. For example, in dynamic contexts when performing non-routine tasks, transactive memory systems moderate the relationship between implicit coordination and adaptive behaviours [47]. This means that, when teams are fully aware of who knows what within the team, the positive effect of implicit coordination processes on performance is more pronounced.

3.3 Teams as complex adaptive systems (CAS)

Since Arrow, McGrath and Berdahl [48] characterised teams as complex adaptive systems (CAS), multiple theoretical frameworks have emerged to capture and explain this idea. However, relatively few empirical studies have been able to examine how long it takes teams to become effective and how these effects develop over time [49–51]. CAS are open systems that are characterised by the level of uncertainty regarding their evolution over time given the interaction of their components [52]. Ramos-Villagrasa et al. [51] carried out a systematic review through the nonlinear dynamical system theory lens, supporting the view of teams as complex adaptive systems. Teams are complex because they are integrated within organisations that exhibit complex behaviour; they are adaptive because they dynamically cope with environmental changes; and they are systems because their functioning depends on the team's history and, therefore, on inputs, but also on the anticipated future, that is, on outputs. The continuous adaptive process that occurs within these teams allows them to adapt to contextual discontinuities and to make decisions according to both the team's antecedents and projected results [48]. The use of this new conceptual approach can help researchers to study teams in a non-linear and more dynamic way [51], as well as to address temporal problems [53, 54] by taking measures at different stages of the team's evolution.

In the case of healthcare teams, they cannot always function as CAS [55]. For example, in clinical situations where problems are identified and described in detail and solutions standardised in specific procedures, teams operate in a planned way, and guidelines are clear and executed in a simple way. However, when there is uncertainty about how to best handle a given situation, operating as a CAS may be the most appropriate option as it promotes the development of new ideas and approaches. This is based on 7 principles: (1) team members can operate autonomously guided by ground rules; (2) team members interact in non-linear ways, i.e., they are interdependent and affect other team members in different ways; (3) the team is sensitive to initial conditions; (4) interactions between team members can produce unpredictable behaviours; (5) these interactions can generate new behaviours; (6) the team is an open system interacting with the environment; and (7) team members function as attractors modelling team behaviour [55].

3.4 Multiteam systems

In the same complex adaptive system stream, teams can be studied from the multiteam system (MTS) perspective [56]. An MTS corresponds to "two or more teams that interface directly and interdependently in response to environmental contingencies toward the accomplishment of collective goals" (p. 289) [56]. These systems constitute "networks of interdependent teams that coordinate at some level to achieve proximal and distal goals" (p. 479) [57]. In a system of this nature, the processes established between the various teams, the cross-team processes, are even more important for the system's success than within-team processes [58]. In the case of the healthcare industry, the use of a multiteam system logic is very beneficial, but much remains to be studied. For example, one area where team research is needed is how best to form networks that integrate patients and their families over time [59]. Patients and their support structures are responsible for coordinating care tasks and helping interpret the information collected, extending beyond the boundaries of healthcare providers. Consequently, managing this extended multi-team system holistically will certainly have very positive results on patient care.

A literature review conducted by Shuffler and Carter [60] identified 7 important lessons for successful teamwork in an MTS: (1) MTS functioning is suited to contexts that are ambiguous, multifaceted, dynamic, and where there is a need for a sense of urgency; (2) MTS structures provide the specialisation, flexibility, and integration needed to deal with complex problems; (3) the teamwork phenomenon changes when moving from a teamwork logic within a team to a teamwork logic within an MTS, for example, cross-team processes take on sovereign relevance; (4) an MTS implies added barriers to collaboration that should be specifically addressed; (5) the incorporation of linking elements can benefit the system's performance; (6) the structure of the MTS and the design of its functioning should be carefully thought out; and (7) leadership plays a crucial role in an MTS and should be integrated and managed across the system [60].

3.5 Facets of team effectiveness

Another relevant framework used to study team effectiveness was suggested by Mathieu et al. [25] illustrating the simultaneous and interrelated relationships among factors associated with team and individual outcomes. Based on a revision of team research published in the *Journal of Applied Psychology* (JAP) during the last century, Mathieu et al. [25] propose a summary construct domain framework with three main facets (**Figure 3**): (a) team task and structure; (b) member characteristics and team composition; and (c) team process and emergent states or mediating mechanisms. This framework captures the many overlapping facets of team effectiveness, providing an in-depth and integrative review of all the constructs that scholars have used thus far to help to advance the teamwork field.

Many of these constructs have been studied among healthcare teams. For example, O'Donovan et al. [62] recently developed a psychological safety measurement instrument designed specifically for healthcare teams. In this instrument, the authors combine the strengths of observation measures with survey measures, allowing for their application to longitudinal studies. Another tool has also been developed to measure the collective intelligence of primary healthcare teams [63]. Collective intelligence can prevent repeating past mistakes and help teams to be more efficient. Jean et al. [63] argue that intelligent teams produce high quality clinical services, so it is essential to better understand the concept and be able to measure it accurately.

Johnson [4] found that intra-team communication demonstrates recurring problems that make it difficult for healthcare teams to coordinate, proposing that teams should work within a common framework represented by formal, informal, market, and professional relationships, or a unique mix based on a mutual orientation towards patient outcomes. The formal approach is based on explicit knowledge and a shared system of codes that, for example, can be translated into written guidelines for hospitals. In addition, the formal approach considers that: personal relationships are also a source of informal information that can overcome the barriers created by formal panels; market logic relates to the creation of information and knowledge-exchange relationships that tend to be maintained through the

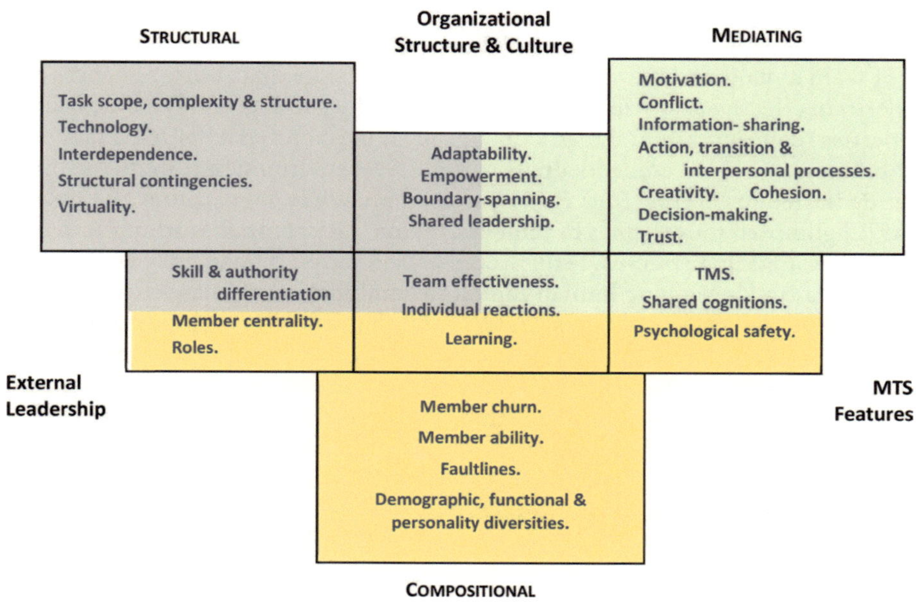

Figure 3.
Facets of the team effectiveness domain based of one century of JAP publications (Source: [61]. Note. MTS = Multiteam Systems. TMS = Transactive Memory System. Some of the constructs overlap dimensions, showing all possible relations between the squares' main facets. These small squares can be seen where coloured squares intersect.)

investment that has been put into the relationship; and professional relationships relate to communication within the domain of professions by creating networks of contacts between professionals based on mutual help. Information-sharing and supportive behaviours have also been observed to have a positive impact on innovation in healthcare teams [64].

A study conducted by Jaca, et al. [65] revealed that the role of the external leader in healthcare teams is quite relevant, and his/her main function is to serve as a team performance coordinator. There is also a clear definition of roles, which facilitates decision-making and conflict management. Furthermore, internal communication and participation levels tend to be high. However, team recognition and training need to be improved, as these are the weakest points in healthcare teams. Several studies have also drawn attention to the importance of teamwork in healthcare and, in particular, the importance of interventions to promote teamwork [3, 66]. One of these types of interventions is "TeamSTEPPS" (Team Strategies and Tools to Enhance Performance and Patient Safety), developed by the Agency for Healthcare Research and Quality (AHRQ) in the USA. TeamSTEPPS is based on communication, leadership, mutual support, and situation monitoring. Another useful model is CRM (Crew Resource Management), which has a significant impact on knowledge and behaviour in acute care settings, such as healthcare [3].

4. Future research avenues

Despite the remarkable advance in team work research, scholars agree on the need for more robust research designs to contribute to the field's further advancement. In addition to the meta-analysis contributions summarizing past empirical findings [17, 18, 67–69], there is consensus among scholars demanding further conceptual frameworks, as well as powerful research designs that capture process-oriented theory and research on team effectiveness [29, 70].

Humphrey and Aime [6] call for a multilevel, multi-theoretical, and multiperiod framework to cope with the contextual dynamics and enhance the understanding of team dynamics. Likewise, Mathieu et al. [30] state that future advances on workgroup effectiveness will be linked with the ability to capture dynamic team properties (conceptually and methodologically); the complexity of team task environments; and the embeddedness in multilevel environments. In the special issue dedicated to *Creating High Performance Teamwork in Organizations*, O'Neil and Salas [2] glimpsed four themes to achieve a team's full potential: working across boundaries; building effective team processes and states; managing team development issues; and leveraging human capital –a combination of knowledge, skills, competences, and other members' and leaders' characteristics. Abrantes et al. [70] highlight 3 types of challenges for research on teams: a theoretical challenge related to team dynamics and the need to identify internal and external drivers that explain these dynamics; a temporal challenge that relates to the process of emergence of team variables and how and when these variables can be assumed to be truly existing phenomena; and a methodological challenge linked to the creation of tools that enable measuring dynamic processes in a non-invasive way. Furthermore, according to Ployhart et al. [71], the agenda for future research on high performance work teams will focus on the conception of teams as adaptive and self-adjusting social entities, embedded in multi-team systems, and as social networks within and outside the team. Therefore, beyond the need to embrace the organizational nature of teams and phenomena at various levels [6], there is also consensus on the need to grasp the dynamic nature of team processes, as they have been assessed primarily as static constructs [26, 29, 70, 72].

As seen, team scholars agree regarding the need for innovative research designs and new techniques to capture team dynamics over time. In this sense, Delice et al. [73] summarize and review existing empirical studies that use novel measurements to study team dynamics over extended periods. Some of these innovative research designs are based on techniques such as role-playing simulations, videotape and software coding, videogames, video-coding, team decision tasks, and whatsApp ICT (information and communication technology). Delice et al. [73] also propose longitudinal laboratory experiments and time-series analyses. Other alternatives include scenario-based studies, critical incident techniques, concept-mapping, cross-border e-business website analyses, and simulations (simulation tasks and longitudinal organizational, computer game-based, and dynamic decision-making simulations), as well as experiential learning approaches and performance assessments, among others. There is, therefore, a plethora of alternatives that should be used to further our understanding of teams that are dynamic and part of adaptive systems [73].

5. Concluding thoughts

In summary, some of the key ideas for future research attempt to overcome the limitations of traditional self-reported assessments, which suffer from problems such as low response rates, response bias, or intrusiveness [29, 74, 75]. Some research strategies that can help to overcome these effects:

- Using more than one measurement method, potentially avoiding single-source bias as well as survey respondent fatigue [26].

- Conceptualizing multiple levels, process dynamics, and the emergence of team phenomena over time [29].

- Increasing the use of measurement technology such as CM-computational modelling, ABBs, etc. [26, 73, 76].

- Addressing and reporting on the different types of work interdependence (task or outcome interdependence) [18].

- Thinking about new ways of obtaining team data such as emails, smartphones, video surveillance, etc., to replace multiple data collection points and traditional self-reported surveys [29].

- At the more conceptual level, possible strategies include:

- Understanding the Multiteam System better as well as team network dynamics in the organizational context [26].

- Bringing the complexity that surrounds modern team-based organizational designs to the fore of team research [70].

Author details

Mercè Mach[1*], António C.M. Abrantes[2] and Ceferí Soler[3]

1 Faculty of Economics and Business, University of Barcelona, Barcelona, Spain

2 ICN Business School – CEREFIGE, Nancy, France

3 ESADE Business School, Ramon Llull University, Barcelona, Spain

*Address all correspondence to: merce.mach@ub.edu

IntechOpen

© 2021 The Author(s). Licensee IntechOpen. This chapter is distributed under the terms of the Creative Commons Attribution License (http://creativecommons.org/licenses/by/3.0), which permits unrestricted use, distribution, and reproduction in any medium, provided the original work is properly cited.

References

[1] Cross, R., Rebele, R., & Grant, A. (2016). Collaborative overload. *Harvard Business Review, 94*,74-79.

[2] O'Neill, T. A., & Salas, E. (2018). Creating high performance teamwork in organizations. *Human Resource Management Review*, *28*(4), 325-331.

[3] Buljac-Samardzic, M., Doekhie, K. D., & van Wijngaarden, J. D. (2020). Interventions to improve team effectiveness within health care: a systematic review of the past decade. *Human Resources for Health, 18*(1), 1-42.

[4] Johnson, J. D. (2019). Framing communication in health care action teams. *International Journal of Healthcare Management, 12*(1), 68-74.

[5] Kozlowski, S. W., & Ilgen, D. R. (2006). Enhancing the effectiveness of work groups and teams. *Psychological Science in the Public Interest*, 7(3), 77-124.

[6] Humphrey, S. E., & Aime, F. (2014). Team microdynamics: Toward an organizing approach to teamwork. *Academy of Management Annals, 8*(1), 443-503.

[7] Carley, K. (1991). A theory of group stability. *American Sociological Review*, *56*, 331-354.

[8] Salas, E., Sims, D. E., & Burke, C. S. (2005). Is there a "big five" in teamwork?. *Small Group Research, 36*(5), 555-599.

[9] Salas, E., Burke, C. S., & Cannon-Bowers, J. A. (2000). Teamwork: emerging principles. *International Journal of Management Reviews, 2*(4), 339-356.

[10] McGrath, J. E. (1984). *Groups: Interaction and performance* (Vol. 14). Englewood Cliffs, NJ: Prentice-Hall.

[11] Stewart, G. L., & Barrick, M. R. (2000). Team structure and performance: Assessing the mediating role of intrateam process and the moderating role of task type. *Academy of Management Journal*, *43*(2), 135-148.

[12] Lehmann-Willenbrock, N., & Allen, J. A. (2018). Modeling temporal interaction dynamics in organizational settings. *Journal of business and psychology*, *33*(3), 325-344.

[13] Lehmann-Willenbrock, N., & Allen, J. A. (2014). How fun are your meetings? Investigating the relationship between humor patterns in team interactions and team performance. *Journal of Applied Psychology, 99*(6), 1278-1287.

[14] Mohammed, S., Ferzandi, L., & Hamilton, K. (2010). Metaphor no more: A 15-year review of the team mental model construct. *Journal of Management, 36*(4), 876-910.

[15] Santos, C. M., Uitdewilligen, S., & Passos, A. M. (2015). A temporal common ground for learning: The moderating effect of shared mental models on the relation between team learning behaviours and performance improvement. *European Journal of Work and Organizational Psychology, 24*(5), 710-725.

[16] Maynard, M. T., Kennedy, D. M., & Sommer, S. A. (2015). Team adaptation: A fifteen-year synthesis (1998 – 2013) and framework for how this literature needs to "adapt" going forward. *European Journal of Work and Organizational Psychology, 24*(5), 652-677.

[17] Gully, S. M., Incalcaterra, K. A., Joshi, A., & Beaubien, J. M. (2002). A meta-analysis of team-efficacy, potency, and performance: Interdependence and level of analysis as moderators of

observed relationships. *Journal of Applied Psychology, 87*(5), 819-832.

[18] Courtright, S. H., Thurgood, G. R., Stewart, G. L., & Pierotti, A. J. (2015). Structural interdependence in teams: An integrative framework and meta-analysis. *Journal of Applied Psychology, 100*(6), 1825-1846.

[19] Bachrach, D. G., Powell, B. C., Collins, B. J., & Richey, R. G. (2006). Effects of task interdependence on the relationship between helping behavior and group performance. *Journal of Applied Psychology, 91*(6), 1396-1405.

[20] Kiggundu, M. N. (1981). Task interdependence and the theory of job design. *Academy of Management Review, 6*(3), 499-508.

[21] Thompson, J. D. (1967). *Organizations in Action*. New York: McGraw Hill.

[22] *D'Silva, J. L., Ortega, A., & Sulaiman, A. H. (2016). Influence of personal and task interdependence on task conflict and team effectiveness. Modern Applied Science, 10(4), 95-100.*

[23] Steiner, I. D. (1972). *Group process and productivity* (pp. 393-422). New York: Academic press.

[24] Mohammed, S. N., Mathieu, J. E., & Bartlett, A. L. (2002). Technical administrative task performance, leadership task performance, and contextual performance: Considering the influence of team- and task-related composition variables. *Journal of Organizational Behavior, 23*, 795-814

[25] Mathieu, J. E., Hollenbeck, J. R., van Knippenberg, D., & Ilgen, D. R. (2017). A century of work teams in the Journal of Applied Psychology. *Journal of Applied Psychology*, *102*(3), 452-467.

[26] Salas, E., Reyes, D. L., & McDaniel, S. H. (2018). The science of teamwork: Progress, reflections, and the road ahead. *American Psychologist*, *73*(4), 593-600.

[27] Hackman, J. R., & Morris, C. G. (1975). Group tasks, group interaction process, and group performance effectiveness: A review and proposed integration. *Advances in Experimental Social Psychology*, *8*, 45-99.

[28] McGrath, J. E. (1964). *A social psychological: A brief introduction*. New York. NY: Holt Rinehart and Winston.

[29] Kozlowski, S. W., & Chao, G. T. (2018). Unpacking team process dynamics and emergent phenomena: Challenges, conceptual advances, and innovative methods. *American Psychologist,* 73, 576-592.

[30] Mathieu, J. E., Wolfson, M. A., & Park, S. (2018). The evolution of work team research since Hawthorne. *American Psychologist, 73*(4), 308-321.

[31] Marks, M. A., Mathieu, J. E., & Zaccaro, S. J. (2001). A temporally based framework and taxonomy of team processes. *Academy of Management Review, 26*(3), 356-376.

[32] *Forsyth, D. R. (2010). Group dynamics.* Belmont, CA: Wadsworth.

[33] Ilgen, D. R., Hollenbeck, J. R., Johnson, M., & Jundt, D. (2005). Teams in organizations: From input-process-output models to IMOI models. *Annual Review of Psychologhy*, *56*, 517-543.

[34] Rico, R., Sánchez-Manzanares, M., Gil, F., & Gibson, C. (2008). Team implicit coordination processes: A team knowledge–based approach. *Academy of Management Review, 33*(1), 163-184.

[35] Mathieu, J. E., Luciano, M. M., D'Innocenzo, L., Klock, E. A., & LePine, J. A. (2020). The development and construct validity of a team processes survey measure.

Organizational Research Methods, *23*(3), 399-431.

[36] Grossman, R., Friedman, S., & Kalra, S. (2017). Teamwork processes and emergent states. In E. Salas, R. Rico, & J. Passmore (Eds.), *The wiley blackwell handbook of the psychology of team working and collaborative processes* (1st ed., pp. 245-269). John Wiley & Sons.

[37] Abrantes, A. C. M., Mach, M., & Ferreira, A. I. (2020). Tenure matters for team cohesion and performance: the moderating role of trust in the coach. *European Sport Management Quarterly*, 1-22.

[38] Mach, M., Dolan, S., & Tzafrir, S. (2010). The differential effect of team members' trust on team performance: The mediation role of team cohesion. *Journal of Occupational and Organizational Psychology, 83*(3), 771-794.

[39] Ahronson, A., & Cameron, J. E. (2007). The nature and consequences of group cohesion in a military sample. *Military Psychology, 19*(1), 9-25.

[40] Carron, A. V. (1982). Cohesiveness in sport groups: Interpretations and considerations. *Journal of Sport Psychology, 4*(2), 123-138.

[41] Charbonneau, D., & Wood, V. M. (2018). Antecedents and outcomes of unit cohesion and affective commitment to the Army. *Military Psychology, 30*(1), 43-53.

[42] Fulmer, C. A., & Gelfand, M. J. (2012). At what level (and in whom) we trust: Trust across multiple organizational levels. *Journal of Management, 38*(4), 1167-1230.

[43] Mayer, R. C., Davis, J. H., & Schoorman, F. D. (1995). An integrative model of organizational trust. *Academy of Management Review, 20*(3), 709-734.

[44] Mohammed, S., Hamilton, K., Tesler, R., Mancuso, V., & McNeese, M. (2015). Time for temporal team mental models: Expanding beyond "what" and "how" to incorporate "when". *European Journal of Work and Organizational Psychology, 24*(5), 693-709.

[45] Austin, J. R. (2003). Transactive memory in organizational groups: The effects of content, consensus, specialization, and accuracy on group performance. *Journal of Applied Psychology, 88*(5), 866-878.

[46] Wegner, D. M. (1995). A computer network model of human transactive memory. *Social Cognition, 13*(3), 319-339.

[47] Marques-Quinteiro, P., Curral, L., Passos, A. M., & Lewis, K. (2013). And now what do we do? The role of transactive memory systems and task coordination in action teams. *Group Dynamics: Theory, Research, and Practice, 17*(3), 194-206.

[48] Arrow, H., McGrath, J. E., & Berdahl, J. L. (2000). *Small groups as complex systems: Formation, coordination, development, and adaptation*. Thousand Oaks, CA: SAGE.

[49] Devaraj, S., & Jiang, K. (2019). It's about time – A longitudinal adaptation model of high-performance work teams. *Journal of Applied Psychology, 104*(3), 433-447.

[50] Kozlowski, S. W. J., & Bell, B. S. (2003). Work groups and teams in organizations. In W. C. Borman, D. R. Ilgen, & R. J. Klimoski (Eds.), *Handbook of psychology (Vol 12): Industrial and organizational psychology* (pp. 333-375). New York: Wiley

[51] Ramos-Villagrasa, P. J., Marques-Quinteiro, P., Navarro, J., & Rico, R. (2018). Teams as complex adaptive systems: Reviewing 17 years of research. *Small Group Research*, *49*(2), 135-176.

[52] Guastello, S. J., & Liebovitch, M. (2009). Introduction to nonlinear dynamics and complexity. In S. J. Guastello, M. Koopmans & D. Pincus (Eds.), *Chaos and complexity in psychology: The theory of nonlinear dynamical systems* (pp. 1-40). New York, NY: Cambridge University Press.

[53] McGrath, J. E., Arrow, H., & Berdahl, J. L. (2000). The study of groups: Past, present, and future. *Personality and Social Psychology Review, 4*, 95-105.

[54] Navarro, J., Roe, R. A., & Artiles, M. I. (2015). Taking time seriously: Changing practices and perspectives in work/organizational psychology. *Revista de Psicología del Trabajo y de las Organizaciones, 31*, 135-145.

[55] Pype, P., Mertens, F., Helewaut, F., & Krystallidou, D. (2018). Healthcare teams as complex adaptive systems: understanding team behaviour through team members' perception of interpersonal interaction. *BMC Health Services Research, 18*(1), 1-13.

[56] Mathieu, J. E., Marks, M. A., & Zaccaro, S. J. (2002). *Multiteam systems.* In N. Anderson, D. S. Ones, H. K. Sinangil, & C. Viswesvaran (Eds.), *Handbook of industrial, work and organizational psychology, Vol. 2. Organizational psychology* (p. 289-313). Sage Publications, Inc.

[57] Zaccaro, S. J., Dubrow, S., Torres, E. M., & Campbell, L. N. (2020). Multiteam systems: An integrated review and comparison of different forms. *Annual Review of Organizational Psychology and Organizational Behavior*, 7, 479-503.

[58] Marks, M. A., DeChurch, L. A., Mathieu, J. E., Panzer, F. J., & Alonso, A. (2005). Teamwork in Multiteam Systems. *Journal of Applied Psychology, 90*(5), 964-971.

[59] Weaver, S. J. (2016). From teams of experts to mindful expert teams and multiteam systems. *Journal of Oncology Practice, 12*, 976-979.

[60] Shuffler, M. L., & Carter, D. R. (2018). Teamwork situated in multiteam systems: Key lessons learned and future opportunities. *American Psychologist, 73*(4), 390-406.

[61] Construct domain for team research. Reprinted from "A century of work teams in the Journal of Applied Psychology" by J. E. Mathieu, J. R. Hollenbeck, D. van Knippenberg, and D. R. Ilgen, 2017, Journal of Applied Psychology, p. 456. Copyright, 2017, by the American Psychological Association

[62] O'Donovan, R., Van Dun, D., & McAuliffe, E. (2020). Measuring psychological safety in healthcare teams: developing an observational measure to complement survey methods. *BMC Medical Research Methodology, 20*(1), 1-17.

[63] Jean, E., Perroux, M., Pepin, J., & Duhoux, A. (2020). How to measure the collective intelligence of primary healthcare teams?. *Learning Health Systems, 4*(3), e10213.

[64] Moser, K. S., Dawson, J. F., & West, M. A. (2019). Antecedents of team innovation in health care teams. *Creativity and Innovation Management, 28*(1), 72-81.

[65] Jaca, C., Viles, E., Tanco, M., Mateo, R., & Santos, J. (2013). Teamwork effectiveness factors in healthcare and manufacturing industries. *Team Performance Management: An International Journal, 9*(3/4), 222-236.

[66] West, M. A., & Lyubovnikova, J. (2013). Illusions of team working in health care. *Journal of Health Organization and Management, 27*(1), 134-142.

[67] LePine, J. A., Piccolo, R. F., Jackson, C. L., Mathieu, J. E., & Saul, J. R. (2008). A meta-analysis of teamwork processes: Tests of a multidimensional model and relationships with team effectiveness criteria. *Personnel Psychology, 61*(2), 273-307.

[68] Schmutz, J. B., Meier, L. L., & Manser, T. (2019). How effective is teamwork really? The relationship between teamwork and performance in healthcare teams: A systematic review and meta-analysis. *BMJ open, 9*(9), e028280.

[69] Stewart, G. (2000). Meta-analysis of work teams research published between 1977 and 1998. *Academy of Management Proceedings* (Vol. 2000, 1, pp. 1-1). Briarcliff Manor, NY 10510: Academy of Management.

[70] Abrantes, A. C. M., O'Neill, T. A., & Passos, A. M. (2020). A temporal perspective on teams. In *Handbook on the Temporal Dynamics of Organizational Behavior* (pp. 274-289). Edward Elgar Publishing.

[71] Ployhart, R.E., Nyberg, A.J., Reilly, G., & Maltarich, M.A. (2014). Human capital is dead; long live human capital resources! *Journal of Management, 40*(2), 371-398.

[72] Mathieu, J. E., Gallagher, P. T., Domingo, M. A., & Klock, E. A. (2019). Embracing complexity: Reviewing the past decade of team effectiveness research. *Annual Review of Organizational Psychology and Organizational Behavior*, 6, 17-46.

[73] Delice, F., Rousseau, M., & Feitosa, J. (2019). Advancing teams research: What, when, and how to measure team dynamics over time. *Frontiers in Psychology, 10*, 1324.

[74] *Feitosa, J., Grossman, R., & Salazar, M. (2018). Debunking key assumptions about teams: The role of culture. American Psychologist, 73(4), 376-389.*

[75] Golden, S. J., Chang, C. H., and Kozlowski, S. W. (2018). Teams in isolated, confined, and extreme (ICE) environments: Review and integration. *Journal of Organizational Behavior, 39*, 701-715.

[76] Kozlowski, S. W., Chao, G. T., Grand, J. A., Braun, M. T., & Kuljanin, G. (2016). Capturing the multilevel dynamics of emergence: Computational modeling, simulation, and virtual experimentation. *Organizational Psychology Review*, *6*(1), 3-33.

Chapter 4

Spiritual Environment Management Tool

Maria Joelle

Abstract

This chapter is about the spiritual environment management tool, which includes spirituality at work and spiritual practices. This management tool is divided into two steps: diagnostic of the worker's perceptions about spirituality at work (first step) and spiritual practices design (second step). By meaning, spirituality at work can help healthcare managers to build effective teamwork in medicine. Spirituality at work has a multidimensional and measurable nature and is aligned with the three principles of the World Health Organization, based on two arguments: the new approach should be preventive and should promote partnership. This fact allows the managers as well the human resource department to classify the organizational environment on the next spiritual issues in the first step: meaningful work; opportunities for inner life; the sense of community; alignment with the organization's value; emotional balance and inner peace. The reduction of medical errors to improve patient safety require the performance of multistep tasks of the great complexity of healthcare professionals, and this chapter pretends to show how the spiritual environment management tool can contribute with the "all working together" goal through a multi-disciplinary care team.

Keywords: teamwork, healthcare, spiritual environment, management tool, well-being

1. Introduction

The purpose of this chapter is to contribute with the concern of this book: the need for a multi-disciplinary care Team - all working together - to help coordinate and optimize the care of patients with complex medical problems.

Can the development of a spiritual environment to help with this concern? This chapter pretends to answer this question and to demonstrate how can spiritual environment as a management tool to help healthcare professionals.

It's very important to contextualize this concept to help us understand how its implementation can contribute to the effective creation of teamwork in healthcare.

Spirituality at work approach is aligned with the principles of different international organizations [1], and the academic evidence shows us, that this approach is useful as a management tool, guiding healthcare practitioners.

The world can be defined as an organization's society, and the scientific community has the responsibility to explain the power and the role of organizations for the achievement of the well-being of the society as a whole.

Spirituality at work has a multidimensional nature, and is aligned with the next three principles of the World Health Organization:

I. The work should be performed in a safe and healthy environment

II. The work conditions should be consistent with the well-being and human dignity

III. The work should provide individual achievement and service for the whole society

The '60s represent a decade in which emerges the consciousness of the negative impacts of the organizational practices on the workers' health and well-being. Attending to this fact, the World Health Organization, appealed to define new perspectives that inspire a positive organizational behavior based on two arguments: these new perspectives should be preventive; and the new human resources policies should promote authenticity, trust, and partnership.

The World Health Organization refers precisely both globalization and technological advance as the two big drivers in the labor world transformation, opening opportunities for a dangerous global competition, looking for financial results in detriment of fundamental human rights and well being.

The new developing technologies and the internet came to show that the line that separates professional and private life became almost invisible and work-life balance became questioned. The stress from this new reality during the XXI century influences negatively the workers' physical and mental health causing absenteeism, low motivational levels, satisfaction and creativity decrease, and organizational productivity and competitiveness reduction. In other words, we are facing conditions that are globally a concern to us all, that represent serious social and financial costs.

Currently, we are facing with weakened economy healthcare and a rapidly changing and increasingly high-tech environment, which requires healthcare workers more contact with screens than with patients [2]. The same authors claim that during these times of high burnout and low engagement levels, the healthcare workers feel the need to bring their whole selves to the work. Please, take note of the previous expression: "whole selves to the work"!

Work environments with a superior spiritual environment have higher individual and organizational outcomes, both within and outside of the healthcare industry [1–3]. So, we are facing the moment to establish the connection between the spiritual environment and the need for a multi-disciplinary care Team - all working together - to help coordinate and optimize the care of patients with complex medical problems.

Exist a connection between spirituality and organization, which is easily established after a deep analysis of the spirituality at work concept and its impacts on the improvement of attitudes and individual performance at work (**Figure 1**), as we will see next. To establish this connection and answering all inheriting concerns related to conceptualization and measurement, a dialog was established between spirituality and science, accepting the Maslow's idea [3]:

"I want to demonstrate that spiritual values have naturalistic meaning, that they are not the exclusive possession of organizational churches, that they are well within the jurisdiction of a suitable enlarged science, and that, therefore they are the general responsibility of all mankind".

This responsibility mentioned in the previous paragraph has been assumed in social sciences by several authors, where the search for the "naturalistic meaning"

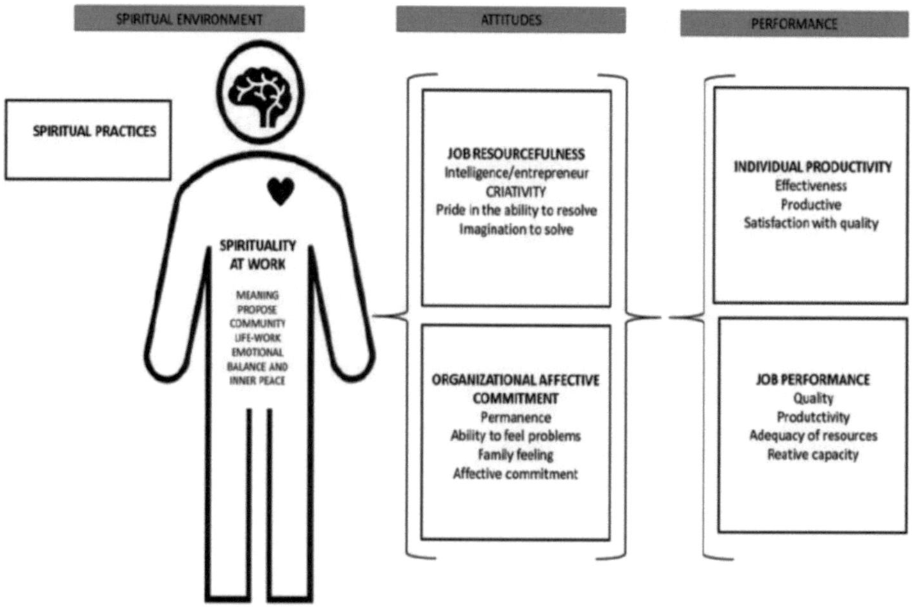

Figure 1.
Spiritual environment. Source: Developed by the author.

is guided by organizational excellence, looking for an organizational purpose or humanitarian aid [4, 5].

The presence of spirituality at work is related to several concerns that should be familiar to leaders, as values and integrity, as the contribution to society, as to take care and support, and as being true [6]. The same authors refer that spirituality at work is both organizational and individual concerns. That is, the leaders need to value the spirituality in their own lives to develop this approach as an organizational management tool, and they will play a role differentiator inside organizations where they belong.

So, spiritual leadership is about creating meaning and value for people, in work life, family life, or community life, as a person who inspires others, promoting higher levels of workforce engagement with their jobs and organizations [4].

The spiritual leadership is related to workplace spiritual intelligence attribute, and both can improve lower levels of job stress, higher levels of workforce engagement, that is greater motivation to improve performance [5].

If the hottest buzz [7] is about the triple bottom line (3 P), a commitment with people, planet, and profit, this buzz should be aligned with another triple bottom line (3 E): employees, environment, and economic.

We need, together, think and act about the importance of both 3 P and 3 E.

So, the humankind needs an evolution more healthy. If we need a more healthy planet/environment, if we need a solid profit/economy, we need healthy people/employees too. And the work, in this complex world, can play a vital role, through a spirit-team-at-work.

So, can we survive without the wealth professionals? Can the world survive without them? We need them. The world needs you! And, we must not forget: you are employees and human beings first!

We can state that health professionals have the mission to supports the pains of humanity. Which is not easy! It is here that spirituality at work emerges as a management tool, as suggested by several authors [1, 2, 7] described in the next section.

2. Teamwork and spiritual environment

This section brings us to a series of doubts and questions which will be addressed in the next subsections:

- What defines spirituality at work?
- How to create a spiritual environment?
- Does spirituality at work contribute to improving the workers' well-being and to create effective teamwork?

2.1 Spirituality at work concept

In the year 2000 spirituality at work met a shift mark, with the research developed by the authors Ashmos and Duchon [8] setting the conceptual frontiers and measurement, therefore enabling the research of the spiritual impacts on workers′ attitudes and work-related outcomes. Their initial investigation was published in the Journal of Management Inquiry, based on previous theoretical developments, their conceptualization and measurement inspired most of the subsequent investigations. Spirituality at work has been explored as a multidimensional concept, mainly due to the work of the authors mentioned above. They have been considered the first authors to produce a serious approach to spirituality at work [9–13].

Spirituality at work is not about religion [14] conversion or about getting people to accept a specific belief system [1, 3, 15] and "has taken many forms" [14] (p.80). It is primarily identified with an open mind and involves connectedness [9] and with the connection between others and the workplace environment, and it is related to self-actualization [10].

Spirituality at work is the recognition that workers perform work with meaning and purpose, for them and society as a whole, including a strong sense of enjoyment at work. The workers can find an opportunity at work to express many aspects of one's being, not just the ability to perform physical or intellectual tasks, and they feel work as a source of spiritual growth and connection with coworkers.

In the organizational level spirituality at work is the link between personal values and the organization's mission and purpose, and the source of employee's emotional balance and inner peace. When organizations introduce spirituality at work, it means that they take care of both the mind and spirit of their employees, finding a more holistic picture of the human being [8]. Returning to Maslow's theory of needs, self-actualization and self-transcendence imply the valence of the individual mind and spirit involved in the work component.

If Maslow created the roots and produced the seminal work that showed the importance and gave rise to the spirituality concept on the organizational field, the authors Ashmos and Duchon developed the basic boundaries of the concept and its measurement, giving place to the most significant developments in this field.

The next figure (**Figure 1**) show us the fundamental words which be part of a spiritual environment. The spiritual environment includes five dimensions and spiritual practices. The same figure includes spirituality at work impacts: job resourcefulness (ability and imagination to solve; intelligence), organizational affective commitment (family feeling), individual productivity (effectiveness), and job performance (quality, relative capacity).

The previous figure (**Figure 1**) shows spirituality at work as a multidimensional concept defined by the next five dimensions:

- Meaningful work involves a deep sense of meaning and purpose in one's work, for workers and society as a whole including the sense of contribution to the community (items related to work that coincides with personal life values and is helpful for the community) and sense of enjoyment at work (items related to a sense of joy and pleasure at work).
  The work can be a way to understand the meaning of life.
  Meaningful work happens when people experience a deep sense of meaning when they perform their work. People have an intrinsic drive and motivation to learn and find meaning in their work and to be a member of a group, where they feel valued for their contribution to the group's performance [11].

- Opportunities for inner life is about finding an opportunity at work to express many aspects of one's being.
  Opportunities for inner life measures the degree to which organizations respect the spiritual values of the workers [12] and was identified by the authors Ashmos and Duchon [8] as spiritual identity: "an opportunity at work to express many aspects of one's being, not merely the ability to perform physical or intellectual tasks" (p.136).
  Spirituality at work begins by acknowledging that people have an inner and outer life, and inner life exists when workers find their inner strengths and use them to perform their tasks at work.

- A sense of community or sense of connection between workers is a human goal at work because although money is important it is not the most important goal for most people. A sense of community is described as the feeling of connectedness that workers develop with other coworkers.
  A sense of community represents another fundamental dimension to create effective teamwork because people want to feel connected to work and they want to feel connected at work [8, 9].
  This concept captures the degree to which employees feel the existence of teamwork connects them as a family in the organization to which they belong, as well as the perception that the supervisors do their best to encourage the presence of effective work.
  A sense of community is described as the feeling of connectedness that workers develop with other coworkers [13], and success can be described using terms such as being connected and balanced.
  The sense of connection is a feeling far beyond oneself, with a genuine sense of community arising from the presence of affections [9].
  Spirituality at work is related to the teamwork concept, once the sense of connection is better understood when we realize meaningful work, and colleagues take the place of family and social groups.

- Alignment with the organization's values is about the personal values and the organization's mission and purpose [16].
  This dimension captures the gap between the workers' perceptions and attitudes and the values of their organizations.
  Alignment with the organization's values measures aspects related to the leader's interests, particularly if there are concerns beyond financial issues. Issues as the perceptions about the organization's future, the way that workers inner life and peace are respected, and finally, the leadership's attitudes to society. These issues are fundamental to create effective teamwork.

- Emotional balance and inner peace capture the emotional balance and inner peace at an individual level when workers perform meaningful work, as explained above. This dimension reinforces the coherence of the overall spirituality at work concept and covers these aspects already anticipated by Maslow [3, 15, 17], and to enrich the traditional approaches of spirituality at work and reinforce the overall coherence of the concept, currently based on four dimensions: inner life, meaningful work, sense of community and values alignment. Emotional balance and inner peace are related to the importance of the happiness that can be felt through work, allowing to find a feeling of inner peace and emotional balance when something goes wrong [1]. With this dimension, we can create a clear connection between the individual and organizational levels, since employees with higher welfare and better life balance are stronger and more persevering [15].

2.2 The link between spirituality at work and teamwork

Through analysis of Maslow's Theory of Needs, a reason was found to establish a link between spirituality at work and organizations [18]. So to begin the understanding about this link, we need to remember the following question, built by Maslow on September 14, 1967, in San Francisco, where he delivered a public lecture titled "The farther reaches of human nature":

- "What are the moments which give you ... the greatest satisfaction? What are the moments of reward which make your work and your life worthwhile?"

The answer to the previous question can be contextualized through the updated version of the Maslow's hierarchy, that includes the next six motivational levels [18]:

- Physiological (survival needs) – seeks to obtain basic needs to survive

- Safety needs – seeks security

- Belongingness and love needs – seeks affiliation with a group

- Esteem needs – seeks esteem trough recognition or achievement

- Self-actualization – seeks fulfillment of personal potential

- Self-transcendence – seeks to a cause beyond the self and to experience communion beyond the boundaries of the self through peak experience

Maslow's studies created the foundations of the spirituality at work concept, identifying the dimensions to the self-actualization and self-transcendence [17]: unique self, peak experience and transcendence, spirituality and meaning, and esthetic-creative element.

Maslow gave an additional contribution to helping the launch in 1969 of the Journal of Transpersonal Psychology, and several other specialists found there a good opportunity to clarify the spirituality at work concept and the role of spirituality may have in the organizational context, in the management, and leadership fields [17].

This new approach contributes to a natural commitment to actions related to justice, trust, beauty, order, simplicity, meaning, and purpose [17]. It is important to note that self-actualizing people are committed with themselves and with the well-being of their groups and community [17] when they are committed whit these intangible being-values [3].

Many academic studies give us insights about how a spiritual environment can help organizations increase their performance and improve the link between workers, between workers and the organization. And, both the self-actualization need and the self-transcendence need, are related to spirituality, and more specifically, related to spirituality inside organizations.

As Maslow explained a self-actualizing person can transcend to individual concerns when he/her being feels actualizing. And these individual concerns are related to intrinsic willingness to serve others, devotion to an ideal, or involvement with a cause as social justice. The self-transcendence person can become relatively egoless. So, to be self-actualizing is not enough for a full description of the human being.

This description of the human being leads us to the words of Chattopadhyay [4]: good people management is more important than all other factors since organizations need to create a work environment that helps them attract, keep and motivate the workers. Dr. (Prof) Debaprasad Chattopadhyay reinforces the idea stating that "the creation of challenge and meaningfulness for employees has become a priority" and "how individuals within organizations can maintain inner and outer balance is an important issue" (p.75).

A multi-disciplinary care team - all working together - to help coordinate and optimize the care of patients with complex medical problems, as mentioned before, meaning effective teamwork, that can reduce medical errors, improving patient safety, requires good people in the management. The presence of spirituality at work can help, since can represent the link between the concern of this book with the words of Dr. (Prof) Debaprasad Chattopadhyay.

How spirituality can help health professionals? Spirituality at work can help them by making organizations socially responsible [7] what includes: the impacts on the environment, the impacts on the community, and the possibility to create a better world. Once, spirituality at work look at people not only as human resources but as whole human beings, including their spiritual needs [19] helping workers "become a spiritual being on a human journey" [17] p.747. And, spiritual leadership is about identifying and affirming shared core values, vision, and purpose with meaning for everybody; meaningful work and community [4].

3. Spiritual environment implementation

The Institute of Medicine (IOM) identified six key measures to improve the overall quality of the healthcare system: safety, effectiveness, patient-centeredness, timeliness, efficiency, and equity [20]. The balanced pursuit of these six key measures is not easy with the current challenges facing by healthcare organizations, as well as other organizations belonging to other industries.

Rational common interests and rational individual interests conflict [20] frequently, and this issue does not promote effective teamwork.

The academic research shows us some evidence which justified the relationship between teamwork and patient safety [21]: investigations about the factors contributing to critical incidents and adverse events have shown that teamwork plays an important role in the causation and prevention of adverse events; some studies focusing on healthcare providers' perceptions of teamwork demonstrated that staff's perceptions of teamwork and attitudes toward safety-relevant team behavior were related to the quality and safety of patient care, and perceptions of teamwork and leadership style are associated with staff well-being, which may impact clinician' ability to provide safe patient care; observational studies on teamwork behaviors related to high clinical performance have identified patterns of communication, coordination, and leadership that support effective teamwork.

The creation and implementation of a spiritual environment may be one strategic imperative of the new millennium, once "people with heart" are "good people management", and good people management is more important than other organizational factors [4]. A spiritual environment includes spiritual practices and spirituality at work [22], as we can see in **Figure 1**, and in this subsection, we will address the implementation.

In the introduction of this chapter, was asked to note the expression "whole selves to the work". This expression helps us to understand the importance of the spiritual environment for healthcare professionals, to bring their whole selves to their organizations where they belong.

The spiritual environment as a management tool can have a positive impact on the development of a care team, with the natural meaning of this concept as claimed by Maslow. Even as create an environment where workers may find meaning in their lives, resilience to overcome obstacles upon fulfilling a fundamental human need [23].

A solid healthcare system requires a healthy work environment, with the compassion feeling between workers as between workers and patients, so the workers need to perform their tasks where the expression "whole selves to the work" is a priority. And we cannot forget: they support all the pain of the humankind. They represent the hope for those who suffer from the most varied pathologies.

The author Pfeffer [24] (p.32) noted four dimensions that workers seek in the workplace:

1. A kind of work that permits to learn and develop a sense of competence and mastery

2. Meaningful work that provides some feeling of purpose

3. A sense of connection and positive social relations with their coworkers

4. The ability to live an integrated life, so that one's work role and other roles are not inherently in conflict and so that a person's work role does not conflict with his or her essential nature and who the person is as a human being

True spiritual leadership enables workers to find these four dimensions, through a training program about a shared spiritual environment, which includes both spiritual practices and spirituality at work concept.

The first step should be diagnostic and measure the level of spirituality at work through the five dimensions previously described, which include 22 questions. This first step allows us to know the organization about the presence of spirituality at work. That is, it allows us to answer the question:

- Have the healthcare professionals the recognition that they have an inner life that nourishes and is nourished by meaningful work that takes place in a community context, with a sense of alignment between individual and organizational values with a sense of emotional balance and inner peace?

After the diagnostic, the next step (second step) should be the development of spiritual practices to implement a spiritual environment.

The implementation of spiritual programs in the workplace can have results at the individual level contributing to the multi-disciplinary care team. Corporate programs and spiritual practices should be custom-designed and adapted to the individuality, values, and perspectives of the workers [25].

Academic studies identified a set of spiritual practices: fitness relaxation practice, meditation, reiki, health programs, hygiene and food education, yoga, pilates, dance, diversity support programs, and music [1].

All these spiritual practices benefit health and well-being and are reported in various investigations in the areas of psychology and health. These different practices may contribute to the development of a sense of community within the team, alignment with organizational values, meaningful work, opportunities for the inner life, and emotional balance and inner peace. And this impacts explained why the practices mentioned called by "spiritual practices" can contribute with the goal "all working together".

4. Conclusion

In the introductory chapter "Medical Error and Associated Harm - The Critical Role of Team Communication and Coordination" of the book "Vignettes in Patient Safety" the authors claim that "the focus on patient safety has its genesis in the combined desire and duty to "do the right thing" in conjunction with the realization that there is an unacceptably high prevalence of avoidable adverse events, we must all join forces and make the effort to meaningfully contribute at the personal, team, and institutional levels" [26]. We find here words and issues which by natural meaning are connected with the spiritual management tool, supporting the link between spirituality at work concept and effective teamwork.

Many researchers emphasize the importance of spirituality at work within organizations, and this growing interest among academics, managers, and the general public [27]. This approach can be seen as a new paradigm change inside the academic context and management thinking.

In recent years, research using diverse methodological approaches has led to significant progress in teamwork research in healthcare [21]. This chapter explained the spiritual environment management tool concept and how can contributes to the creation of a multi-disciplinary care team - all working together - to help coordinate and optimize the care of patients with complex medical problems.

To achieve collective prosperity through work, the International Labor Organization considers fundamental values as freedom, human dignity, social justice, security, and non-discrimination. The spiritual environment is aligned with these values as well as principles of the World Health Organization.

Spiritual environment, can play a fundamental role in healthcare organizations since spirituality at work is definable and measurable, and the inclusion provides intrinsic and extrinsic reasons as organizational affective commitment, job resourcefulness [22], and organizational performance [9, 28].

Attending the spirituality at work concept, a spiritual environment is created when the companies respect cultural diversity and personal values of workers by implementing employee development programs, employee participation in the decision, and healthy employer-employee relations [14]. The implementation of spiritual programs can boost results at the individual level, such as self-efficacy, greater willingness to cooperate, grow, learn, and adapt to challenges [1, 25, 27].

The spiritual practices should respond to organizational and individual concerns as explained in Subsection 2.2. To create a spiritual environment a greater consensus is required to move the whole organization.

Author details

Maria Joelle
Polytechnic Institute of Coimbra, Coimbra, Portugal

*Address all correspondence to: mariajoelle7@gmail.com

IntechOpen

© 2020 The Author(s). Licensee IntechOpen. This chapter is distributed under the terms of the Creative Commons Attribution License (http://creativecommons.org/licenses/by/3.0), which permits unrestricted use, distribution, and reproduction in any medium, provided the original work is properly cited.

References

[1] Joelle M, Coelho A. The impact of a spiritual environment on performance mediated by job resourcefulness. *Int J Work Heal Manag*; 12. Epub ahead of print 2019. DOI: 10.1108/IJWHM-05-2018-0058.

[2] Doram K, Chadwick W, Bokovoy J, et al. Got spirit? the spiritual climate scale, psychometric properties, benchmarking data, and future directions. BMC Health Serv Res. 2017;**17**:1-7

[3] Wulff DM, Maslow AH. Religions, Values, and Peak-Experiences. J Higher Educ. 1965;**36**:235

[4] Chattopadhyay, Debaprasad. Case Study Spiritual Motivation in Management : A Case Study on how Spirituality in Management can be used by a health-care provider *** " SGCC & RI - A big leap in the service to Mankind". 2016; 74-87.

[5] Roberts G. Leadership coping skills: Servant leader workplace spiritual intelligence. J Strateg Leadersh. 2013;**4**:52-69

[6] Smith JA, Rayment JJ. The Global SMP fitness framework: A guide for leaders exploring the relevance of spirituality in the workplace. Manag Decis. 2007;**45**:217-234

[7] McLaughlin C. Spirituality and ethics in business. Eur Bus Rev. 2005;**17**:236-243

[8] Ashmos DP, Duchon D. Spirituality at Work: A Conceptualization and Measure. J Manag Inq. 2000;**9**:134-145

[9] Daniel JL. Workplace spirituality and stress: Evidence from Mexico and the US. Manag Res Rev. 2015;**38**:29-43

[10] Deshpande AR. Workplace Spirituality, Organizational Learning Capabilities, and Mass Customization: An Integrated Framework. Int J Bus Manag. 2012;**7**:3-18

[11] Milliman J, Czaplewski AJ, Ferguson J. Workplace spirituality and employee work attitudes: An exploratory empirical assessment. J Organ Chang Manag. 2003;**16**:426-447

[12] Rego A, Pina E, Cunha M. Workplace spirituality and organizational commitment: An empirical study. J Organ Chang Manag. 2008;**21**:53-75

[13] Joelle M, Coelho A. Adding a new dimension to the spirituality at work concept: Scale development and the impacts on individual performance. Manag Decis. 2019;**58**:982-996

[14] Gupta M, Kumar V, Singh M. Creating Satisfied Employees Through Workplace Spirituality: A Study of the Private Insurance Sector in Punjab (India). J Bus Ethics. 2014;**122**:79-88

[15] Sanders JE, Hopkins WE, Geroy GD. From Transactional to Transcendental: Toward An Integrated Theory of Leadership. J Leadersh Organ Stud. 2003;**9**:21-31

[16] Milliman J, Ferguson J. In Search of the 'Spiritual' in Spiritual Leadership: A Case Study of Entrepreneur Steve Bigari. Bus Renaiss Q. 2008;**3**:19

[17] O'connor D, Yballe L. Maslow revisited: Constructing a road map of human nature. J Manag Educ. 2007;**31**:738-756

[18] Koltko-Rivera ME. Rediscovering the later version of Maslow's hierarchy of needs: Self-transcendence and opportunities for theory, research, and unification. Rev Gen Psychol. 2006;**10**:302-317

[19] e Cunha MP, Rego A, D'Oliveira T. Organizational Spiritualities. Bus Soc 2006; 45: 211-234.

[20] Berwick DM, Nolan TW, Whittington J. The triple aim: Care, health, and cost. Health Aff. 2008;**27**:759-769

[21] Manser T. Teamwork and patient safety in dynamic domains of healthcare: A review of the literature. Acta Anaesthesiol Scand. 2009;**53**:143-151

[22] Joelle M, Coelho AM. The impact of spirituality at work on workers' attitudes and individual performance. Int J Hum Resour Manag. 2019;**30**:1111-1135

[23] Yeoman R. Conceptualising Meaningful Work as a Fundamental Human Need. J Bus Ethics. 2014;**125**:235-251

[24] Pfeffer, J.: 2003, 'Business and the Spirit: Management Practices that Sustain Values', in R. A. Giacalone and C. L. Jurkiewicz (eds.), Handbook of Workplace Spirituality and Organizational Performance (M.E. Sharpe, Armonk, NY), pp. 29-45.

[25] Karakas F. Spirituality and performance in organizations: A literature review. J Bus Ethics. 2010;**94**:89-106

[26] Green A, Stawicki S. Firstenberg M. Introductory Chapter: Medical Error and Associated Harm - The Critical Role of Team Communication and Coordination. 2018. DOI: 10.5772/intechopen.78014

[27] Sprik PJ. The Depersonalization of Medicine, and the Promises of Spiritual Care. Society. 2019;**56**:147-152

[28] Brophy M. Spirituality Incorporated: Including Convergent Spiritual Values in Business. J Bus Ethics. 2015;**132**:779-794

Chapter 5

Learning Health-Care Worker Networks from Electronic Health Record Utilization

You Chen

Abstract

The health-care system is a highly collaborative environment where health-care workers collaborate to care for patients. Health-care organizations (HCOs) design and develop various types of staffing plans to promote collaboration among health-care workers. The existing staffing plans describe the cooperation at a coarse-grained level, such as team scheduling. They seldom consider connections among health-care workers and investigate how health-care workers receive and disseminate information, which is essential evidence to inform actionable staffing interventions to improve care quality and patient safety. In this chapter, we introduce how to apply network analysis methods to electronic health record (EHR) utilization data to learn connections among health-care workers and build networks to describe teamwork in a fine-grained level. The chapter includes: (i) a brief description of the EHR utilization data, (ii) approaches to learn connections among health-care workers, (iii) building health-care worker networks, (iv) developing survey instruments to validate health-care worker networks, (v) introducing sociometric measurements to quantify network structures and positions of health-care workers in the networks, (vi) using statistical models to test associations between teamwork structures and patient outcomes, and (vii) listing examples to learn health-care worker networks in an HCO and a specific setting, including neonatal intensive care unit and trauma.

Keywords: network analysis, methodology, collaboration, care team, patient outcome, electronic health record, data-driven, data mining, bottom-up, health-care worker network, health-care organization, sociometric measurement, audit logs, statistical model, survey instrument, network structure

1. Introduction

The United States health-care system has been moving to patient-centered care by incorporating different levels of collaborations, including those occurring within a health-care organization (HCO) or between HCOs [1, 2]. A classic model [3] proposed to understand patient-centered care divides the health-care system into four nested levels: (1) the individual patient; (2) the care team made up of health-care workers (e.g., clinicians, pharmacists, social workers, and utilization managers) to care for patients; (3) the HCO (e.g., hospital, clinic, and nursing home) that supports the development and work of care teams by providing infrastructure and complementary resources; and (4) the political and economic

IntechOpen

environment (e.g., regulatory, financial, payment regimes, and markets) that support hospital collaborations with other HCOs and payers on population health management. To promote patient-centered care, HCOs create infrastructures and develop staffing strategies to encourage collaboration among health-care workers to care for patients [4, 5]. Collaboration among health-care workers can improve care quality (e.g., reducing readmission rates) [6], patient safety (e.g., preventing medical errors) [7], and patient outcome (shortening length of stay) [8–10].

Staffing plans describe collaboration at a macro-level. For instance, an intensive care unit (ICU) may use an intensivist-centered care team (closed model) or an ad hoc group consisting of nurses, nurse practitioners, and physicians (open model) to care for critically ill patients [11]. The macro-level staffing strategies seldom specify how health-care workers connect and how they receive and disseminate information to care for patients. Thus, it is difficult for HCOs to monitor those top-down staffing strategies implemented in clinical practice. Without the micro-level knowledge of teamwork (e.g., health-care worker connection), it is challenging for HCOs to assess their staffing strategies to identify inefficient and ineffective parts for further collaboration optimization.

Measuring connections among health-care workers is very challenging due to complex clinical workflows and dynamic structures of teamwork [12, 13]. That is also one of the reasons why HCOs do not specify connections among health-care workers in their staffing plans. Recent studies show connections among health-care workers can be learned from their activities in electronic health record (EHR) systems [14–19]. EHR systems are a platform used by health-care workers to diagnose patients and exchange diagnostic results [20, 21]. In modern health-care environments, an increasing number of health-care workers utilize EHR systems as the primary tool to diagnose patients and exchange health information [22]. Therefore, the volume and scale of the EHR system utilization data have been increasing exponentially in recent years, which provide abundant resources for researchers to learn collaborations through the EHR system utilization [14–19].

In this chapter, we provide a network analysis of the EHR system utilization data to learn teamwork structures and specify connections among health-care workers. We believe the chapter can provide researchers a new way to model teamwork/collaboration in health care. We anticipate the data, methods, and applications introduced in this chapter will be of interest to the teamwork in health-care readership, particularly those focused on network analysis, secondary data analysis, EHR utilization, and care teams.

2. EHR system utilization data

EHR systems provide a platform for care coordination across a diverse collection of health-care workers [22–25]. Coordination activities occurring in EHR systems play an increasingly important role in the establishment of high-efficient health-care worker collaboration networks. Various studies, including our prior research, have leveraged health-care worker activities in EHR systems to infer patterns of collaboration [9, 10, 14–19]. The proportion of care activities performed via EHR systems has steadily increased with the adoption of EHR through meaningful use of incentives [22, 26].

Health-care worker activities occurring in EHR systems have been documented in the form of audit logs. When a provider accesses or moves between modules in the EHR interface, such as moving from Progress Notes to Order Entry, a record of these activities are documented, including the time the event occurred, the health-care worker and patient IDs, and the computer location. Audit logs include all health-care worker interactions to EHRs of patients, which provides an opportunity to study connections among health-care workers. The continuous data collection of the EHR audit logs provides robust, readily available data. Since health-care worker activity is documented in the EHR in near real time, it is free from recall bias and variation introduced when health-care workers are retrospectively surveyed to describe their activities in EHRs.

The activities performed by health-care workers stem from six primary sources [10], including conditions (e.g., assigning a diagnosis), procedures (e.g., intubation), medications (e.g., prescription), notes (e.g., progress note writing), orders (e.g., laboratory test ordering), and measurements (e.g., measuring respiratory rate).

Figure 1 shows an example to illustrate health-care worker activities in EHR systems. Each event, such as *requesting a lab test*, includes a health-care worker, an EHR, and the time stamp. The four events depicted in the example demonstrate the hidden collaborations between health-care workers. For instance, the physician ordered a lab test and shared the order with the lab user; next, the lab user conducted the laboratory test and shared the test results of the patient with a health-care worker in the physician office; finally, the nurse practitioner reviewed and analyzed the results.

3. Transforming utilization data into matrices

Events document interactions of health-care workers to EHRs of patients, but they do not capture the direct connections among health-care workers. As shown in **Figure 1**, the four health-care workers performed events to EHRs of a patient, and they are not directly connected. We leverage events to measure the hidden connections among health-care workers. A hidden connection between two health-care workers is defined based on their interactions with the EHRs of patients. We call a hidden connection as an indirect relationship, because the two health-care workers do not communicate directly, but care for the same patients via performing actions to their EHRs. For instance, a physician ordered a lab test and sent the order to a

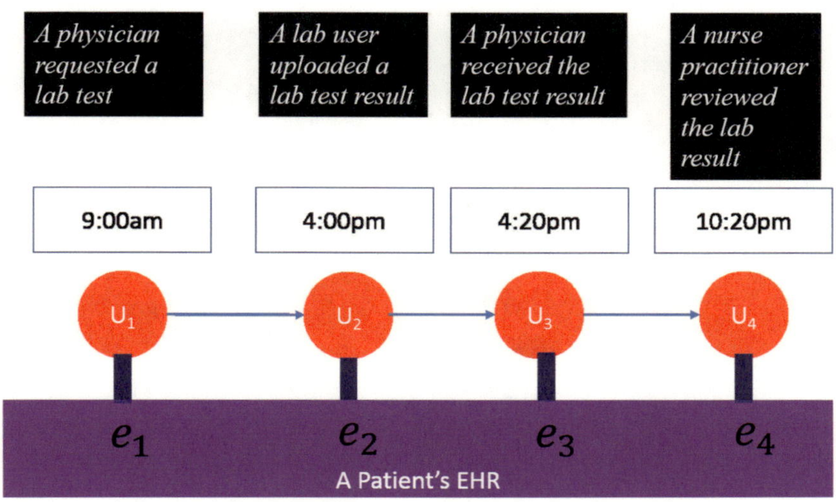

Figure 1.
An example to illustrate data elements in EHR audit logs. Four health-care workers performed their actions to EHRs of a patient at different time stamps on the same day.

laboratory test user. The physician and the lab user have a hidden relationship that is built upon the lab test order. Hidden relations are essential knowledge to characterize processes of health information sharing and dissemination among health-care workers in EHR systems, which can potentially impact teamwork, and the following care quality and patient safety.

We use a bipartite graph of EHR users (health-care workers) and EHRs of subjects (patients) to represent events a user performed to EHRs of a subject. **Figure 2** shows an example of a bipartite graph, and a binary matrix to characterize interactions of six users to EHRs of seven subjects. In the example depicted in the figure, we use a binary matrix to represent if a health-care worker performed events to EHRs of a subject within a period (e.g., hour, day, week, or length of stay). Researchers can determine the period and whether using a binary value or the number of events to represent interactions of a health-care worker with EHRs of a patient according to their research purpose. To simplify our process, we use a binary matrix *A*, as shown in **Figure 2**. As mentioned above, if two health-care workers performed events to EHRs of the same patients within a period (e.g., a day), then there exists a hidden relationship between them. For instance, u_1 and u_3 both performed events to EHRs of s_1 and s_2. Thus, in the binary matrix, $A(1,1)$, $A(1,3)$, $A(2,1)$, $A(2,3)$ are all ones. To transforming health-care works' interactions to EHRs to connections among health-care workers, we use binary matrix multiplication. For instance, the relationship between u_1 and u_3 can be learned by multiplying matrix *A* and its transpose matrix *AT*. The results of matrix multiplication are shown in matrix *B* in **Figure 3**. $B(1,3)$ or $B(3,1)$ represents the number of subjects whose EHRs were managed by both u_1 and u_3. From **Figure 2**, we can see the number of subjects co-managed by both u_1 and u_3 is 2, which is equal to $B(1,3)$ or $B(3,1)$. The larger the cell values in matrix *B*, the more strength of the relationship between health-care workers.

Matrix *A* represents the interactions of health-care workers to EHRs of subjects, and *B* describes the relationships between health-care workers. We show a simple way (matrix multiplication) to learn *B* from *A*. There are many alternative or advanced approaches that can be applied to matrix A (binary or nonbinary version) to measure hidden relationships between health-care workers. Examples of such methods include term-frequency, inverse documentary frequency (TF-IDF) [27], principal component analysis (PCA) [28], and similarity measurements

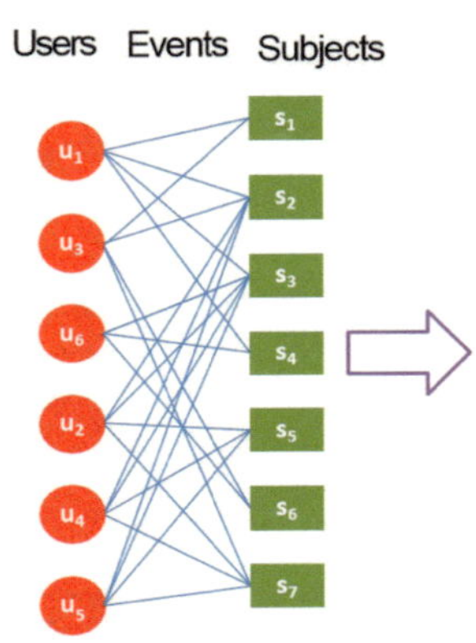

Bipartite graph of users and subjects

	u_1	u_2	u_3	u_4	u_5	u_6
s_1	1	0	1	0	0	0
s_2	1	1	1	1	1	0
s_3	1	1	0	1	1	1
s_4	1	0	0	0	0	1
s_5	0	1	0	1	1	0
s_6	0	0	1	0	0	1
s_7	0	1	1	1	1	0

Binary matrix A of subjects and users

Figure 2.
Events performed by health-care workers (u_i) to EHRs of patients (s_j) are represented by a bipartite graph (left) and corresponding binary matrix (right). In the right subfigure, if a health-care worker, u_i, performed events to EHRs of a patient, s_j, then the cell value $A(i,j)$ in the matrix will be 1, otherwise 0.

DOI: http://dx.doi.org/10.5772/intechopen.93703

	u_1	u_2	u_3	u_4	u_5	u_6
s_1	1	0	1	0	0	0
s_2	1	1	1	1	1	0
s_3	1	1	0	1	1	1
s_4	1	0	0	0	0	1
s_5	0	1	0	1	1	0
s_6	0	0	1	0	0	1
s_7	0	1	1	1	1	0

Binary matrix A

AA^T ⇒

	u_1	u_2	u_3	u_4	u_5	u_6
u_1	4	2	2	2	2	2
u_2	2	4	2	4	4	1
u_3	2	2	4	2	2	1
u_4	2	4	2	4	4	1
u_5	2	4	2	4	4	1
u_6	2	1	1	1	1	3

User-User matrix B

Figure 3.
Using the product of binary matrix A and the transpose matrix AT to calculate the number of subjects whose EHRs are managed by a pair of users. Each cell value B(i,i) in the diagonal represents the number of subjects whose EHRs are managed by u_i. Each cell value B(i,j) $(i \neq j)$ represents the number of subjects whose EHRs are co-managed by both u_i and u_j.

(e.g., cosine, Kullback-Leibler (KL) divergence, edit distance, and Jaccard distance) [29]. For instance, if the size of the matrix is big (a large number of subjects or health-care workers), we can apply PCA to it to reduce the dimensionality first, and then measure relationships for pairs of health-care workers based on the principal components.

4. Building networks

4.1 Relationship measurement

There are two types of relationships: directed and undirected between health-care workers. Directed relation emphasizes on the ordered relations, for instance, the connections from health-care worker A to B, and B to A that are different. To learn directed connection from the utilization data, we use time stamps of events to describe the ordered relationships. As shown in **Figure 1**, lab test ordering occurred ahead of lab test results uploading. Thus, the relationship between the physician who ordered the lab test and the lab user who uploaded the test results is directed. Upon the directed relations, we can create direct networks. We will use an example to illustrate the creation of directed networks of health-care workers concerning the management of each patient. Examples of undirected networks are used to describe structures of collaborations among health-care workers within a unit or across a HCO.

4.2 Directed health-care worker networks

As mentioned above, we define actions performed by a health-care worker in EHR systems as events. Events affiliated with EHRs of a patient constitute a sequence of information flow. We provide a simple scenario to understand the series of information flow as follows.

"The night respiratory therapist documents an increased need for oxygen in a patient's EHRs" → *"the daytime nurse documents the patient's vital signs and notes that the patient has tachypnea"* → *"on rounds the nurse practitioner and attending review the recorded vital signs focusing on the need for more oxygen and elevated respiratory rate"* → *"the physician prescribes a diuretic."*

In this example, the nurse practitioner and attending's comprehension of the patient's condition grew with each update to the EHR. Health-care workers depend on their colleagues to provide information for clinical updates as they are essential to health-care workers' decision-making. As mentioned above, we call this virtual worker-worker interaction a hidden connection. A hidden connection does not mean a face-to-face interaction occurred, but rather, there existed the potential for the neighboring health-care workers to directly exchange information on the patient's condition via the EHR and arrive at the same conclusion, which in this scenario was to prescribe medication for pulmonary edema. We build networks that represent the hidden connections facilitating the dispersion of patient-related information. We call them patient-level health-care worker networks because they are composed of all health-care workers that treated a common patient.

To start, we create a simplified sequence dataset by condensing consecutive events by the same health-care worker into a single event. In this scenario, we can filter the self-loop relationships of health-care workers. In a network or a graph, a self-loop relationship is an edge that connects a vertex/node to itself. For example, health-care worker W_1 made three EHR events consecutively to EHRs of a patient, and we condensed them into one event; one could interpret the simplified sequence as a workflow in EHR. Based on the sequences, we identified relationships between health-care workers whenever their events occurred consecutively (health-care worker W_2 used the patient's EHR after health-care worker W_1). We characterized each hidden connection with the frequency by which they occurred.

Figure 4 shows an example of how we build a health-care worker network from a patient's sequence. As shown in **Figure 4**, the health-care worker W_1 interacted with the EHR before health-care worker W_2, so the arrowhead on the right points to health-care worker W_2. The edge weight is the number of times the hidden interaction occurred. Note an edge exists if an interaction occurred at least once. While an observed interaction was not guaranteed to be an exchange of information, it did have the potential to be one.

4.3 Undirected health-care worker networks: care for a group of patients

The structure of teamwork learned from a single patient is hard to represent the pattern of collaboration concerning the management of a group of patients. In this section, we introduce the creation of undirected health-care workers for the management of a group of patients. We assume health-care workers participating in the care of the same patients (performed events to EHRs of the same patients) on the same day have a relationship. Based on such an assumption, we can create a binary matrix (as shown in **Figure 3**) to describe whether a health-care worker performed events to EHRs of a patient. The cell value 1 is for Yes, and 0 for No. Based on the binary matrix of health-care workers and EHRs of patients, we can use the matrix multiplication, as shown in **Figure 3**, to get the daily relationships between pairs of

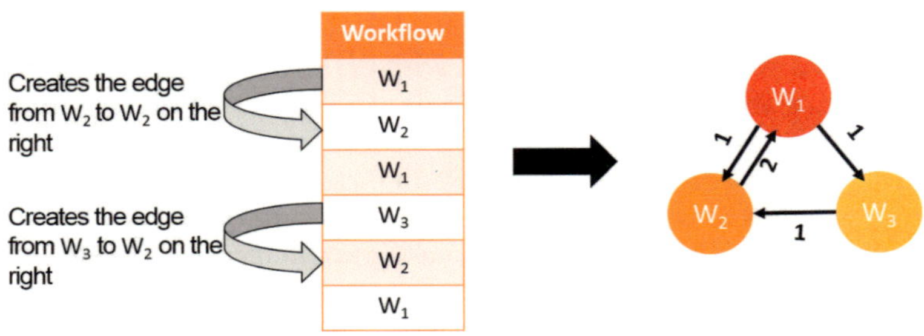

Figure 4.
An example to learn a health-care worker network from a patient's EHR sequence.

health-care workers. Each non-diagonal cell value shows the number of patients; any two health-care workers both performed events to their EHRs on the same day. Two factors determine the strength of the relationship between two health-care workers. The first is the number of patients the two workers performed events to their EHRs on the same day, and the second is the number of days when the two workers performed events to EHRs of the same patients. We build a health-care worker network for a group of patients by using the relationships which are cumulatively added based on the number of days and patients.

We use a simple scenario to explain health-care worker networks built upon a group of patients. Assuming a medical intensive care unit (MICU) adopted a new scheduling strategy in a pandemic (e.g., COVID-19), and the health-care organization plans to investigate the changes in the structure of collaboration among health-care workers before and after the adoption of the new scheduling strategy. In this scenario, we use 8 months (4 months before and after adopting the new scheduling strategy) of EHR utilization data to learn the changes. To implement the study, we create two groups: critically ill patients admitted to the MICU before and after the new scheduling strategy adopted. To ensure the studied two groups share similar confounding factors (e.g., demographics and health conditions), we can use propensity score matching to create them. We use events performed by health-care workers to EHRs of the two groups of patients to measure relationships between health-care workers before and after the adoption of the scheduling strategy, respectively. Based on the relationships, we can build two health-care worker networks: before and after the adoption of the new scheduling strategy. The differences in the structures of the two networks can be measured using sociometric measurements, which are introduced in the following sections.

4.4 Undirected health-care worker networks: care for patients within an HCO

When learning a collaboration network at the level of a health-care organization, the number of patients and health-care workers investigated will be much bigger, and the relationships between health-care workers will become more complex. If we have a large number of patients, then it may complicate the measuring of the relationships between health-care workers. For instance, if we investigate 10,000 health-care workers and 1,000,000 patients, then the size of the health-care worker-patient matrix is 10 K by 1 M. There is a necessity to reduce the dimensionalities of the matrix to ensure it is appropriate for the following approaches to measure relationships between health-care workers. As mentioned above, PCA can be applied to the matrix to reduce dimensionalities. After the dimensionality reduction, we can use similarity measurements (e.g., cosine similarity or KL divergence) to calculate the relationships between health-care workers, which are used to build networks of health-care workers. If PCA is unable to represent the variance of the data in the matrix, an alternative way is to transform the matrix of health-care workers and patients into a higher level. Instead of building networks of health-care workers, we can create networks of operational areas (e.g., medical intensive care unit, and burn center). Also, we can cluster patients into groups according to their phenotypes and transform the matrix of health-care workers by patients into operational areas by patient groups. Based on the new transformed matrix, we measure relationships between operational areas and build a collaboration network of operational areas.

Figure 5 shows an example to illustrate the process of transforming interactions between health-care workers and EHRs of patients into interactions of health-care workers to EHRs of groups of patients. Patient groups can be learned by conducting phenotyping algorithms on patient health conditions and demographics. For instance, a typical topic modeling algorithm – Latent Dirichlet Allocation (LDA) can be used to learn topics to represent phenotypes of each patient. Based on the phenotypic topics, patients can be clustered into groups. As shown in **Figure 5**, the transformation from *Apatient × health condition* to *Bpatient × patient group* can be implemented by using LDA.

Figure 6 shows an example to illustrate the process of transforming interactions between health-care workers and EHRs of patient groups into the interactions between operational areas and EHRs of patient groups, which are further leveraged to measure relationships between operational areas. The transformation from *Dhealth-care worker × patient group* and *Eoperational area × health-care worker* into *Foperational area × patient group* is implemented using matrix multiplication. *Eoperational area × health-care worker* represents the affiliations of health-care workers to operational areas. Similarity measurements can be applied to *Foperational area × patient group* to learn relationships between pairs of operational areas *Roperational area × operational area*. Collaboration networks of operational areas can be built upon the *Roperational area × operational area*. To learn stable relationships between operational areas, we may need to create the matrix *Chealth-care*

$A_{\text{patient} \times \textit{health condition}}$

	c_1	c_2	c_3	c_4	c_5	c_6
p_1	1	0	1	0	0	0
p_2	0	1	0	1	0	0
p_3	1	0	1	0	0	0
p_4	0	1	0	1	0	0
p_5	0	0	0	0	1	1
p_6	0	0	0	0	1	1

$B_{\textit{patient} \times \textit{patient group}}$

	g_1	g_2	g_3
p_1	1	0	0
p_2	0	1	0
p_3	1	0	0
p_4	0	1	0
p_5	0	0	1
p_6	0	0	1

$C_{\text{healthcare worker} \times \textit{patient}}$

	p_1	p_2	p_3	p_4	p_5	p_6
w_1	1	1	0	0	0	0
w_2	0	1	0	0	0	0
w_3	0	0	1	1	0	0
w_4	0	0	0	1	0	0
w_5	0	0	0	0	1	1
w_6	0	0	0	0	0	1

$D_{\textit{healthcare worker} \times \textit{patient group}}$

	g_1	g_2	g_3
w_1	1	1	0
w_2	0	1	0
w_3	1	1	0
w_4	0	1	0
w_5	0	0	2
w_6	0	0	1

Figure 5.
An example to illustrate the process of transforming the interactions between health-care workers and EHRs of patients (Chealth-care worker × patient) into interactions between health-care workers and EHRs of patient groups (Dhealth-care worker × patient group).

$E_{\text{operational area} \times \textit{healthcare worker}}$

	w_1	w_2	w_3	w_4	w_5	w_6
o_1	1	1	0	0	0	0
o_2	1	0	0	0	0	0
o_3	0	0	1	1	0	0
o_4	0	0	0	0	1	0
o_5	0	0	0	0	0	1

×

$D_{\textit{healthcare worker} \times \textit{patient group}}$

	g_1	g_2	g_3
w_1	1	1	0
w_2	0	1	0
w_3	1	1	0
w_4	0	1	0
w_5	0	0	2
w_6	0	0	1

$F_{\text{operational area} \times \text{patient group}}$

	g_1	g_2	g_3
o_1	1	2	0
o_2	1	1	0
o_3	1	2	0
o_4	0	0	2
o_5	0	0	1

$R_{\text{operational area} \times \textit{operational area}}$

	o_1	o_2	o_3	o_4	o_5
o_1	1	0.9	1	0	0
o_2	0.9	1	0.9	0	0
o_3	1	0.9	1	0	0
o_4	0	0	0	1	0.7
o_5	0	0	0	0.7	1

Figure 6.
An example to illustrate the process of transforming interactions between health-care workers and EHRs of patient group (Dhealth-care worker × patient group) into relationships between operational areas (Roperational area × operational area).

worker × *patient* by setting a longer window size, such as 1 week/month rather 1 day we used in the previous examples. A study shows it requires at least 4 weeks to get stable relationships between operational areas by using interactions between health-care workers and EHRs of patients [30].

5. Validating relationships among health-care workers learned from the EHR system utilization

Concerns over the trustworthiness of the results of automated learning methods are not limited to the health-care worker network learned in this chapter. Instead, this is a problem that manifests when any knowledge is learned from the secondary analysis of EHR data. Researchers always need to review the knowledge learned from the data for their plausibility. As we mentioned above, the relationships between health-care workers learned from the utilization data are indirect. In other words, they are not explicitly documented by health-care organizations. To use networks built upon such relationships to describe or interpret structures of collaborations among health-care workers, we need to validate the relationships.

To do so, we design and deploy an online survey to assess the plausibility of relationships among health-care workers. **Figure 7** depicts an example of 626

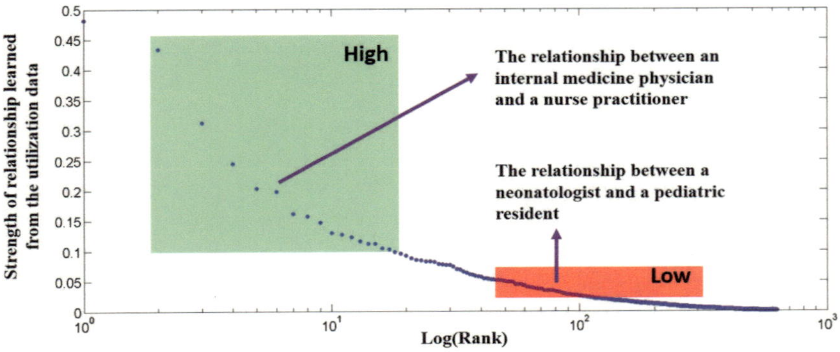

Figure 7.
Relationships between pairs of health-care workers ranked by their strength. Each of the two shaded areas represents relationships with high and low strengths, respectively. Each node in the graph represents a relationship.

relationships ranked on a log scale and the strength of the relationships. This is clearly more relationships than a human can evaluate without fatigue, and so we need to sample a small number of them for respondents to assess. For instance, we can randomly select 20 relationships: 10 of high, and 10 of low strength. A survey can be designed to evaluate a specific hypothesis of the form: hospital employees can correctly distinguish between relationships of high and low strengths.

A survey contains a series of questions. The hospital employees who respond to the survey are presented with questions of the form: "*An internal medicine physician performed actions to the record of patient John Doe. How likely is it that an internal medicine nurse practitioner performed actions to the same patient's record?*". Respondents are not presented with the strength of the relationship between internal medicine physicians and nurse practitioners. The respondents are asked to choose one of five candidate answers: "Not at all likely," "Slightly likely," "Moderately likely," "Very likely," and "Completely likely." In order to conduct a survey analysis through statistical models, we can convert these answers into integer values in the range 1–5 (e.g., "Not at all likely" is mapped to 1).

A set of respondents will answer each question in the survey. We can conduct a pretest to obtain feedback from the experts to refine the surveys and estimate the required number of experts via a power analysis. REDCap, which is a secure web application for building and managing online surveys and databases [31], can be used to implement the online survey. Details of the plausibility validation of the relationships between health-care workers can be found in our previous works [30, 32]. If we can verify with statistical significance that the learned relationships are often in line with the expectations of hospital employees, then we can suggest that collaboration networks of health-care workers, as well as strategies built on such networks, may be reliable and scalable.

6. Sociometric measurements

Sociometric measurements include network- and node-level metrics. The network-level metrics such as size, graph density, reciprocity, triads, average path length, clustering, cohesion and density, core-periphery, centralization, diameter, and K-core are used to characterize the structure of a network; while the node-level metrics such as degree, closeness, betweenness, eigencentrality, and eccentricity are used to describe the characteristics of each node in the network. In this section, we explain those measurements in the health-care worker networks.

6.1 Network-level metrics

Diameter. The diameter is defined as the number of steps in the longest path in the network. There are two types of paths for any two nodes in the network. The first one is the shortest path, which is defined as the smallest number of steps between the two nodes, and the other one is the longest path, which has the largest number of steps between the two nodes. The network diameter is the number of steps between the two nodes, who have the largest number of steps in their longest path. Given two networks of health-care workers, if the diameter of the first one is larger than the second, then the information sharing and dissemination among health-care workers in the first network requires more steps.

Density and cohesion. Graph density is defined as the total number of edges within the network, divided by the number of edges that could exist. The cohesion of a network is described by the diameter and the average path length. The average path length is the average of the steps between all the nodes in the network. The low diameter or low average path length indicates a cohesive network with little clustering. Usually, when density increases, the average path length decreases because high-density network provides many paths along which to connect nodes. Studies show the relationship between density and average path length is nonlinear [33]. Density values above 0.5 indicate networks have many redundant paths between nodes, and it is hard to identify structures of networks [33]. If density values are very low, then there will be no network structures. To learn structures of health-care worker collaboration networks, we may need to prune the networks by using density values (e.g., <0.5). For instance, we can filter edges whose weight strength is low to decrease the density values of networks.

Core-periphery. Core-periphery structures are networks in which there is a group of nodes that are densely connected to one another (the core) and a separate group of nodes loosely connected to the core and loosely connected to each other (the periphery). It is not uncommon to find core-periphery networks in the health-care domain. In the NICU, nurses, neonatologists, and anesthesiologists work in a core network [9]. In contrast, otolaryngology residents, endocrinology physicians, and hematology physicians collaborate in a periphery network [9].

Centralization. The typical calculation of centralization is as: $\sum_{i=1}^{i=n}\left(\max(v_i)-v_i\right)/\left(n^2-3n+2\right)$, where v_i is the centrality score (e.g., degree, betweenness, and closeness) of a node in the network, and n is the total number of nodes in the network [34]. In the centralized network, one or a few people hold a position of power and control in the network. An alternative way to calculate centralization is to measure the standard deviation of the node centrality scores. A large standard deviation indicates a lot of variation in the individual centrality scores, and hence a centralized structure. In contrast, a small standard deviation suggests little variation and hence a decentralized structure. In a network of health-care workers, if we can identify workers with high centrality scores in the centralized network, then we can further investigate how those workers share and disseminate information in the EHR systems. Do they act like broadcasters to reach many health-care workers quickly, or do they act as gatekeepers to slow down the information sharing and dissemination?

Clustering coefficient. A clustering coefficient is a measure of the degree to which nodes in a graph tend to cluster together. The metric can be defined at the network- and health-care worker levels. The network-level clustering coefficient gives an overall indication of the clustering in the network. The network-level clustering coefficient is measured as: $\#of\ closed\ triplets / \#of\ all\ triplets$, where a triplet is three nodes that are connected by either two (open triplet) or three (closed triplet) undirected edges. If a health-care worker network has a high clustering coefficient, then health-care workers are connected in dense pockets of interconnectivity. There are two types of network structures that connect clustered subgroups. The first is the bridge structure, in which the clustered subgroups are connected by bridges (intermediates), and the second one is the centralized structure, in which central health-care workers connect the subgroups.

Reciprocity. Reciprocity is used to characterize the symmetry in relationships between health-care workers. In network science, the reciprocity is measured in direct networks. A typical approach [35] to calculate the network reciprocity is: $\sum_{i\neq j}\left(a_{i,j}-\bar{a}\right)\left(a_{j,i}-\bar{a}\right)/\sum_{i\neq j}\left(a_{i,j}-\bar{a}\right)^2$, where $a_{i,j}$ is one if a link from i to j exists, and 0, otherwise. $\bar{a}=\sum_{i\neq j}a_{i,j}/n\times(n-1)$, where n is the number of health-care workers in the network. If a network has a higher value of reciprocity, then the greater likelihood of health-care workers to be mutually linked in information receiving and dissemination in the network.

K-core. The K-core is a subset of the network, in which each health-care worker within the K-core is connected to at least K other workers. A health-care worker in the K-core sub-network is considered as one of the cores in the whole network.

6.2 Health-care worker-level metrics

Degree. The degree of a health-care worker is the total number of edges connected. The weighted degree is the sum of the weights of connected edges. In the health-care worker network, the weight of an edge can be the strength of the relationship.

Clustering coefficient. The clustering coefficient of a health-care worker is the proportion of connections among their adjacent health-care workers divided by the number of connections that could possibly exist between them. One can think of the clustering coefficient as quantification of how close a health-care worker's neighbors are to be a clique of clinicians (e.g., a small group of clinicians, with shared interests in common patients). A health-care worker with a large clustering coefficient is the one who shares patients with health-care workers who also share patients with each other [9].

Betweenness. The betweenness is defined as the number of shortest paths between two health-care workers that pass through the specific health-care worker. Betweenness refers to whether a health-care worker lies on the path of others who are not directly connected. A health-care worker with a broad skillset could frequently be in a high-betweenness position. For instance, in **Figure 8**, clinicians 2, 3, and 4 have the largest number of shortest paths going through them. Betweenness reflects a health-care worker's access to diverse communication channels about evidence-based practice. A high betweenness worker cares for a wide spectrum of patients.

Eigencentrality. Eigencentrality is used to quantify the influence or leadership of a health-care worker on the collaboration and coordination among health-care workers in the network. A health-care worker with a high eigencentrality is connected to workers who have high eigencentrality. An example of health-care workers with high eigencentrality is shown in **Figure 9**. A high eigencentrality health-care worker acts as a leader in the sharing of patients in the network.

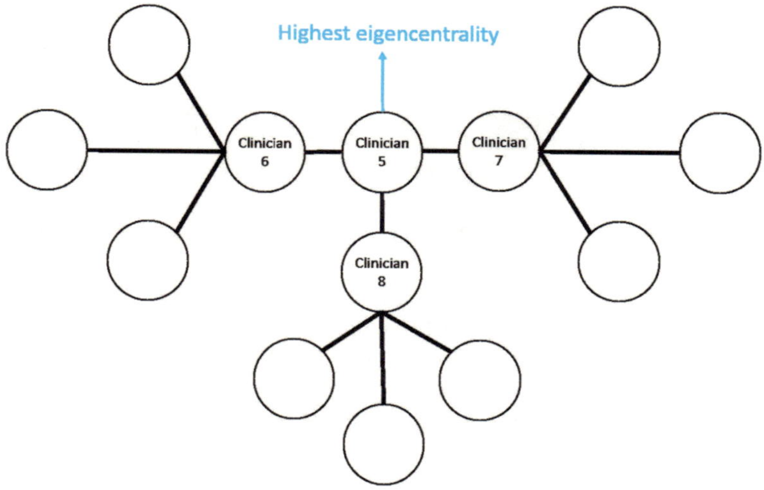

Figure 8.
Examples of health-care workers with the highest betweenness.

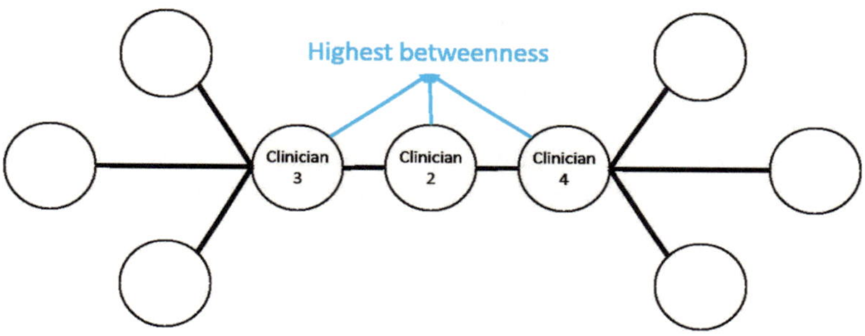

Figure 9.
An example of a health-care worker with the highest eigencentrality.

7. Statistical models to test hypotheses related to network structures

Most of the research studies in health care are hypothesis-driven. One of the goals of the network analysis in health care is to provide evidence on network structure to assist in the designing and development of teamwork-based hypotheses. Various hypotheses can be developed between sociometric measurements and clinical outcomes, including delayed ICU admission, ICU readmission, medication error, adverse event, length of hospital stay (LOS), mortality risk, and health-care cost.

7.1 Relationships of sociometric measurements with clinical outcomes

Structures of teamwork among health-care workers can be quantified by using both network- and node-level sociometric measurements. It has been recognized that structures of teamwork are associated with clinical outcomes. To inform actionable staffing interventions, we can develop hypotheses for each of the sociometric measurements and validate their relationships with clinical outcomes. For each inpatient stay (ranging from their admission to discharge), we can create a network to describe the structure of teamwork among health-care workers during the patient stay. Hypotheses can be designed based on the network. An example of the hypotheses can be: the clustering coefficient of a network is associated with LOS. Statistical models can be leveraged to test the hypotheses. The distributions of most network measurements are not Gaussian distributed, so we can use rank-based approaches to measure associations between the measurements and clinical outcomes. For instance, we can use the Spearman rank-order correlation to measure the association between the clustering coefficient and LOS. If we want to investigate multiple sociometric measurements or add confounding factors (patient demographics, the severity of sickness), we can use advanced statistical models, such as a proportional-odds (PO) logistic regression model.

The PO model can be thought of as a set of logistic regression models, where each model describes the log-odds of LOS (continuous variable) being higher than some threshold j (rather than lower than or equal to), and where $j = 1, 2, \ldots, J$ represents all possible thresholds by which LOS can be dichotomized, and J is equal to the number of unique outcome values minus one. The set of models is collapsed into a single model, via the proportional odds assumption that coefficients for predictor variables are the same across the threshold values. Even when this assumption is not met, a coefficient from the proportional odds model can be thought of as a weighted average of coefficients across all the threshold-specific logistic regression models.

Some outcomes, such as ICU readmission, delayed ICU admission, or mortality risk are categorical variables. In that case, we can use the Mann Whitney U test or analysis of variance (ANOVA) to test the differences in the sociometric measurements between networks. The hypotheses can also be developed between node-level measurements (e.g., betweenness, eigencentrality, and degree) and clinical outcomes. For instance, critically ill patients who were cared for by more high-betweenness nurses were significantly less likely to die in their ICU stays.

7.2 Changes in structures of health-care worker networks

Analyzing changes in the collaboration network structures and measuring relationships of the changes with outcomes are very important research questions in the teamwork in health care. When a health-care organization adopts a new staffing intervention (e.g., creating a new team scheduling), they will need to assess and monitor the changes in the behavior of collaboration among health-care workers before and after the interventions and how such changes impact clinical outcomes. Getting feedback from the adoption of a new staffing intervention can provide evidence to identify weak and ineffective parts to do further optimization. For instance, ICUs adopt staffing interventions in the COVID-19 pandemic, and the responses may change the structure of collaboration. We can use network analysis approaches to analyze the changes in the network structures from pre-COVID-19 to intra-COVID-19 and measure the relationships of such changes with clinical outcomes such as ICU readmission or delayed ICU admission. Examples of hypotheses can be: neonatology physicians have higher betweenness after the staffing intervention or the health-care worker network after the staffing intervention has a larger diameter (the difficulty of sharing patients increases). Since sociometric measurements are not Gaussian distributed in many situations, we can apply a Mann-Whitney U test to measure the significance of the difference.

8. Applications

We introduce three applications to show how we use network analysis to identify care teams in a health-care organization, measure associations between collaborations and length of stay in the trauma setting, and assess health-care worker networks for the management of surgical neonates, respectively.

8.1 Care team identification

We applied network analysis to the EHR utilization records of over 10,000 hospital employees and 17,000 inpatients at a large academic medical center during a 4-month window [19]. The study aimed to learn collaboration structure across the entire health-care system, and thus it built networks of departments (higher level) rather than the networks of health-care workers. Each node in the network is a department. LDA models were used to cluster patients into groups. As shown in **Figures 5** and **6**, matrix multiplications were conducted to transform the matrix of health-care workers and patients into the matrix of departments and patient groups. Connections among 317 departments were inferred from the department-patient group matrix. We identified 34 collaborative groups of departments [19]. Each of the groups is a subnetwork and could be considered as a care team across various types of departments. The results suggested that, although the over 17,000 patients exhibited over 1400 different types of phenotypes, the health-care workers treating them tended to work in only 34 collaborative groups. When the 34 groups were presented to health-care experts via online surveys, 27 (79.4%) of 34 were confirmed as administratively plausible. Of those, 26 teams depicted strong collaborations, with a clustering coefficient >0.5.

8.2 Length of stay and trauma team structures

We started the network analysis of trauma team structures by creating a matrix of ~5000 health-care workers and EHRs of ~5500 patients based on the EHR system utilization data [10]. The difference is we applied a spectral co-clustering methodology to the matrix to infer groups of patients and clusters of health-care workers simultaneously. By using the co-clustering algorithm, we created three trauma patient groups, each of which has a corresponding network of health-care workers. For each network of health-care workers, we calculated sociometric measurements to quantify their structures. Length of stay was used as the outcome. The association between a sociometric measurement (e.g., clustering coefficient) and length of stay was measured by using statistical models incorporating various confounding factors (e.g., demographics and admission dates). We found a remarkably clear distinction in LOS: those patients experiencing the largest quantity of collaborations between health-care workers had the shortest LOS, while those subject to fewer collaborations (i.e., supported by less well-integrated care teams), spent much longer in hospital, indicating greater financial cost as well, of course, as pain, distress, and inconvenience to the patient [10].

8.3 Length of stay and NICU team structures

We extracted EHR data of 15 NICU gastrostomy patients from the day prior to the patient's surgery day until postoperative day 30. The study aims to validate the associations between health-care worker networks and post-surgical length of stay (PLOS) [36]. For each patient ICU stay, we built a directed network to show how information was received and disseminated among health-care workers in the NICU. For each patient's stay, we created a simplified sequence dataset by ordering health-care worker actions based on their time stamps starting from the day prior to the patient's surgery until postoperative day 30 or the patient's discharge date. Based on the sequences, we identified connections between health-care workers whenever their actions occurred consecutively. We learned 15 patient-level health-care worker networks. We used the sociometric measurements, including in-degree, out-degree, and betweenness, to quantify the structures of each patient-level network.

We modeled patient PSLOS with each structure measurement controlling for patient age and weight using a proportional-odds logistic regression model. Study results show health-care workers, whose patients had lower PSLOS, tended to disperse patient-related information to more colleagues within their network than those, who treated higher PSLOS patients ($P = 0.0294$). Our results demonstrate in the NICU that improved dissemination of information may be linked to reduced PSLOS.

9. Conclusions

This chapter provides an introduction of a network analysis of secondary EHR system utilization data to learn health-care worker networks. We introduce five main components when applying network analysis to team structures and clinical outcomes: (i) matrix multiplication to build connection among health-care workers, (ii) survey instruments to validate the plausibility of the learned connections among health-care workers, (iii) sociometric measurements to characterize network structures, (iv) hypothesis development to connect network structures with clinical outcomes, and (v) statistical models to test the hypotheses. Finally, we use three examples to show the application of network analysis in health care. In short, EHR data provide an efficient, accessible, and resource-friendly way to study teamwork using network analysis tools.

Acknowledgements

The research studies introduced in this chapter were supported, in part, by the National Library of Medicine of the National Institutes of Health under Award Numbers K99LM011933, R00LM011933, and R01LM012854.

Conflict of interest

The authors declare no conflict of interest.

Author details

You Chen
Vanderbilt University Medical Center, Nashville, Tennessee, United States

*Address all correspondence to: you.chen@vanderbilt.edu

IntechOpen

© 2020 The Author(s). Licensee IntechOpen. This chapter is distributed under the terms of the Creative Commons Attribution License (http://creativecommons.org/licenses/by/3.0), which permits unrestricted use, distribution, and reproduction in any medium, provided the original work is properly cited.

References

[1] Fix GM, VanDeusen Lukas C, Bolton RE, Hill JN, Mueller N, LaVela SL, et al. Patient-centred care is a way of doing things: How healthcare employees conceptualize patient-centred care. Health Expectations. 2018;**21**(1):300-307

[2] Gusmano MK, Maschke KJ, Solomon MZ. Patient-centered care, yes; patients as consumers, no. Health Affairs. 2019;**38**(3):368-373

[3] Ferlie EB, Shortell SM. Improving the quality of health care in the United Kingdom and the United States: A framework for change. Milbank Quarterly. 2001;**79**(2):281-315

[4] D'Lima DM, Murray EJ, Brett SJ. Perceptions of risk and safety in the ICU: A qualitative study of cognitive processes relating to staffing. Critical Care Medicine. 2018;**46**(1):60

[5] Upadhyay S, Weech-Maldonado R, Lemak CH, Stephenson AL, Smith DG. Hospital staffing patterns and safety culture perceptions: The mediating role of perceived teamwork and perceived handoffs. Health Care Management Review. 25 October 2019. DOI: 10.1097/HMR.0000000000000264. [Epub ahead of print] PMID: 31702706

[6] Newman MW. Integrated and collaborative care: Quality improvement in action. Psychiatric Annals. 2017;**47**(7):374-377

[7] Ma C, Park SH, Shang J. Inter-and intra-disciplinary collaboration and patient safety outcomes in US acute care hospital units: A cross-sectional study. International Journal of Nursing Studies. 2018;**85**:1-6

[8] Reeves S, Pelone F, Harrison R, Goldman J, Zwarenstein M. Interprofessional collaboration to improve professional practice and healthcare outcomes. Cochrane Database of Systematic Reviews. 2017;**6**(6):CD000072

[9] Chen Y, Lehmann CU, Hatch LD, Schremp E, Malin BA, France DJ. Modeling care team structures in the neonatal intensive care unit through network analysis of EHR audit logs. Methods of Information in Medicine. 2019;**58**(4-05):109

[10] Chen Y, Patel MB, McNaughton CD, Malin BA. Interaction patterns of trauma providers are associated with length of stay. Journal of the American Medical Informatics Association. 2018;**25**(7):790-799

[11] Chowdhury D, Duggal AK. Intensive care unit models: Do you want them to be open or closed? A critical review. Neurology India. 2017;**65**(1):39

[12] Rosen MA, DiazGranados D, Dietz AS, Benishek LE, Thompson D, Pronovost PJ, et al. Teamwork in healthcare: Key discoveries enabling safer, high-quality care. The American Psychologist. 2018;**73**(4):433

[13] Jagannath S, Sarcevic A, Marsic I. An analysis of speech as a modality for activity recognition during complex medical teamwork. In: Proceedings of the 12th EAI International Conference on Pervasive Computing Technologies for Healthcare; 21 May 2018. pp. 88-97

[14] Durojaiye AB, Levin S, Toerper M, Kharrazi H, Lehmann HP, Gurses AP. Evaluation of multidisciplinary collaboration in pediatric trauma care using EHR data. Journal of the American Medical Informatics Association. 2019;**26**(6):506-515

[15] Wu DT, Smart N, Ciemins EL, Lanham HJ, Lindberg C, Zheng K.

Using EHR audit trail logs to analyze clinical workflow: A case study from community-based ambulatory clinics. In: AMIA Annual Symposium Proceedings. Vol. 2017. San Francisco, CA: American Medical Informatics Association; 2018. pp. 1820-1827

[16] Amroze A, Field TS, Fouayzi H, Sundaresan D, Burns L, Garber L, et al. Use of electronic health record access and audit logs to identify physician actions following noninterruptive alert opening: Descriptive study. JMIR Medical Informatics. 2019;7(1):e12650

[17] Wang JK, Ouyang D, Hom J, Chi J, Chen JH. Characterizing electronic health record usage patterns of inpatient medicine residents using event log data. PLoS One. 2019;**14**(2):e0205379

[18] Chi J, Bentley J, Kugler J, Chen JH. How are medical students using the electronic health record (EHR)?: An analysis of EHR use on an inpatient medicine rotation. PLoS One. 2019;**14**(8):e0221300

[19] Chen Y, Lorenzi NM, Sandberg WS, Wolgast K, Malin BA. Identifying collaborative care teams through electronic medical record utilization patterns. Journal of the American Medical Informatics Association. 2017;**24**(e1):e111-e120

[20] Durojaiye AB. A novel approach for the investigation of multidisciplinary collaboration using social network analysis on electronic health record data [doctoral dissertation]. Baltimore MD: Johns Hopkins University; 2018

[21] Van Liew JR. Balancing confidentiality and collaboration within multidisciplinary health care teams. Journal of Clinical Psychology in Medical Settings. 2012;**19**(4):411-417

[22] Henry J, Pylypchuk Y, Searcy T, Patel V. Adoption of electronic health record systems among US non-federal acute care hospitals: 2008-2015. ONC Data Brief. 2016;**35**:1-9

[23] Platform IT. Open or closed: A project proposal for investigating two different EHR platform approaches. Context Sensitive Health Informatics: Sustainability in Dynamic Ecosystems. 2019;**265**:207

[24] Ballaro JM, Washington ER. The impact of organizational culture and perceived organizational support on successful use of electronic healthcare record (EHR). Organization Development Journal. 2016;**34**(2):11-29

[25] Serbanati LD, Ricci FL. EHR-centric integration of health information systems. In: 2013 E-Health and Bioengineering Conference (EHB); 21 November 2013. IEEE. pp. 1-4

[26] Adler-Milstein J, Adelman JS, Tai-Seale M, Patel VL, Dymek C. EHR audit logs: A new goldmine for health services research? Journal of Biomedical Informatics. 2020;**101**:103343

[27] Chen K, Zhang Z, Long J, Zhang H. Turning from TF-IDF to TF-IGM for term weighting in text classification. Expert Systems with Applications. 2016;**66**:245-260

[28] Ku W, Storer RH, Georgakis C. Disturbance detection and isolation by dynamic principal component analysis. Chemometrics and Intelligent Laboratory Systems. 1995;**30**(1):179-196

[29] Xuecheng L. Entropy, distance measure and similarity measure of fuzzy sets and their relations. Fuzzy Sets and Systems. 1992;**52**(3):305-318

[30] Chen Y, Nyemba S, Malin B. Auditing medical records access via healthcare interaction networks. In: AMIA Annual Symposium Proceedings. Vol. 2012. American Medical Informatics Association; 2012. p. 93

[31] Harris PA, Taylor R, Minor BL, Elliott V, Fernandez M, O'Neal L, et al. The REDCap consortium: Building an international community of software platform partners. Journal of Biomedical Informatics. 2019;**95**:103208

[32] Chen Y, Lorenzi N, Nyemba S, Schildcrout JS, Malin B. We work with them? Healthcare workers interpretation of organizational relations mined from electronic health records. International Journal of Medical Informatics. 2014;**83**(7):495-506

[33] Friedkin NE. The development of structure in random networks: An analysis of the effects of increasing network density on five measures of structure. Social Networks. 1981;**3**(1):41-52

[34] Freeman LC. Centrality in social networks conceptual clarification. Social Networks. 1978;**1**(3):215-239

[35] Garlaschelli D, Loffredo MI. Patterns of link reciprocity in directed networks. Physical Review Letters. 2004;**93**(26):268701

[36] Kim C, Lehmann C, Schildcrout J, Hatch D, France D, Chen Y. Provider networks in the neonatal intensive care unit associate with length of stay. In: IEEE 5th International Conference on Collaboration and Internet Computing. Los Angeles, CA: IEEE; 2019:127-134

Section 2

Teamwork and Cultures of Safety

Chapter 6

Adverse Events Capture Systems, Checklists and Teamwork as Relevant Tools to Reduce Complications and Increase Patients' Safety in Spinal Surgery

Giovanni Barbanti Brodano, Cristiana Griffoni, Alessandro Ricci, Sandra Giannone, Daniela Francesca Ghisi and Alessandro Gasbarrini

Abstract

Adverse events in Hospitals are often related to surgery and they represent a relevant problem in healthcare. Different approaches have been introduced during the last decade to address the problem of patient safety, especially in the surgical environment. The teamwork is crucial in all these actions which aim to decrease adverse events and improve clinical outcomes. We analyze in particular the use of adverse events capture systems in spinal surgery and the use of checklist systems, starting from the Surgical Safety Checklist introduced by the World Health Organization (WHO) in 2008.

Keywords: adverse events, checklist, outcome, safety, teamwork

1. Introduction

In Hospitals adverse events are not rare. Most of these adverse events are related to surgery. The incidence of surgical complications has remained largely unchanged during the past two decades. Inherent complexity in surgery, new technology possibilities, increasing age and comorbidity in patients may contribute to this. The incidence of surgery-related adverse events combined with the increasing volume of surgery results in a relevant healthcare problem [1].

In a review of adverse events incidence, preventability, and outcome conducted by deVries and co-workers [2], the median incidence rate of adverse events was 9.2% with a probable preventability of 43.5%. Adverse events that led to permanent disabilities were 7%.

The most common surgical complications are related to surgical techniques, infections, and postoperative bleeding [3, 4]. Equipment-related failures contribute to a significant part of errors in the operating room and it has been observed that the use of checklists reduces equipment errors by 48.6 to 60.7% [5].

One of the first large- scale studies on checklists use in healthcare (the Keystone study) was carried out in Michigan in 108 intensive care units, where Provonost and co-workers introduced a series of interventions, including a checklist to improve communications [6]. The intervention reduced venous catheter-related blood-stream infections from 2.7 to 0 after 18 months. However, these results could not be replicated in a large-scale United Kingdom program, revealing a particular attention to the context and implementation strategies in improvement programs [7].

2. The use of surgical safety checklist and other checklist systems

To improve care and safety for surgical patients, a checklist, similar to those used in aviation, aeronautics and product manufacturing, was developed by the World Health Organization (WHO). The Surgical Safety Checklist (SSC) consists of 19 items and it is used at three critical perioperative moments: induction, incision and before the patient leaves the operating room (**Figure 1**). The items contain an oral confirmation by the surgical team of the completion of some key steps necessary to ensure safe delivery of anesthesia, antibiotic prophylaxis, effective teamwork and other essential practices in surgery [8, 9].

Although several investigators have challenged the efficacy of the SSC, it has shown repeated success in reducing preventable intraoperative and postoperative complications, length of hospital stay and overall mortality [10–12]. In addition, the investigators have concluded that the implementation of the SSC in multiple institutions has improved communication, efficiency, and attention to routine details in the operating room.

In a systematic review published on 2014 Bergs and co-workers [10] analyzed the results reported in six studies to assess the effectiveness of the WHO SSC. The results of this meta-analysis suggest that the WHO SSC reduced postoperative complications, including mortality. Meta-analysis demonstrated a significant effect of the checklist on any complication, mortality and surgical site infection. It also suggested that sites with adequate compliance with aspects of patient's care related to the checklist were more likely to demonstrate a significant reduction in postoperative complications. Haynes and colleagues [13] showed that improvements in postoperative outcomes were associated with improved perception of

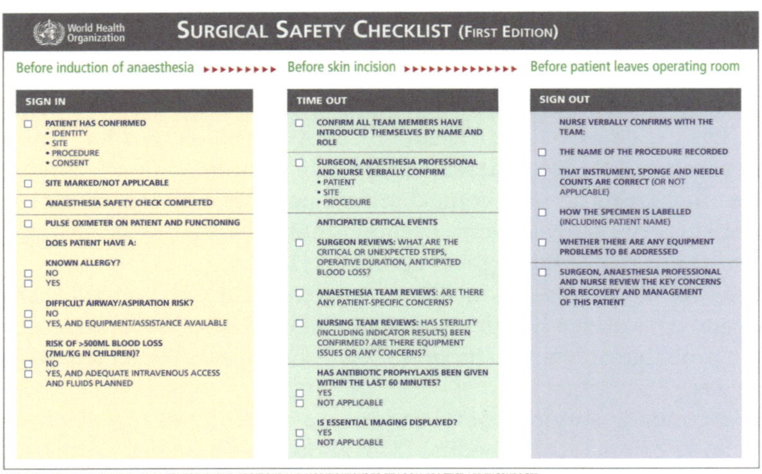
World Health Organization
SURGICAL SAFETY CHECKLIST (FIRST EDITION)

Before induction of anaesthesia ▸▸▸▸▸▸▸▸▸▸ Before skin incision ▸▸▸▸▸▸▸▸▸▸▸▸▸▸ Before patient leaves operating room

SIGN IN

- ☐ PATIENT HAS CONFIRMED
  - IDENTITY
  - SITE
  - PROCEDURE
  - CONSENT
- ☐ SITE MARKED/NOT APPLICABLE
- ☐ ANAESTHESIA SAFETY CHECK COMPLETED
- ☐ PULSE OXIMETER ON PATIENT AND FUNCTIONING

DOES PATIENT HAVE A:

KNOWN ALLERGY?
- ☐ NO
- ☐ YES

DIFFICULT AIRWAY/ASPIRATION RISK?
- ☐ NO
- ☐ YES, AND EQUIPMENT/ASSISTANCE AVAILABLE

RISK OF >500ML BLOOD LOSS (7ML/KG IN CHILDREN)?
- ☐ NO
- ☐ YES, AND ADEQUATE INTRAVENOUS ACCESS AND FLUIDS PLANNED

TIME OUT

- ☐ CONFIRM ALL TEAM MEMBERS HAVE INTRODUCED THEMSELVES BY NAME AND ROLE
- ☐ SURGEON, ANAESTHESIA PROFESSIONAL AND NURSE VERBALLY CONFIRM
  - PATIENT
  - SITE
  - PROCEDURE

ANTICIPATED CRITICAL EVENTS
- ☐ SURGEON REVIEWS: WHAT ARE THE CRITICAL OR UNEXPECTED STEPS, OPERATIVE DURATION, ANTICIPATED BLOOD LOSS?
- ☐ ANAESTHESIA TEAM REVIEWS: ARE THERE ANY PATIENT-SPECIFIC CONCERNS?
- ☐ NURSING TEAM REVIEWS: HAS STERILITY (INCLUDING INDICATOR RESULTS) BEEN CONFIRMED? ARE THERE EQUIPMENT ISSUES OR ANY CONCERNS?

HAS ANTIBIOTIC PROPHYLAXIS BEEN GIVEN WITHIN THE LAST 60 MINUTES?
- ☐ YES
- ☐ NOT APPLICABLE

IS ESSENTIAL IMAGING DISPLAYED?
- ☐ YES
- ☐ NOT APPLICABLE

SIGN OUT

NURSE VERBALLY CONFIRMS WITH THE TEAM:
- ☐ THE NAME OF THE PROCEDURE RECORDED
- ☐ THAT INSTRUMENT, SPONGE AND NEEDLE COUNTS ARE CORRECT (OR NOT APPLICABLE)
- ☐ HOW THE SPECIMEN IS LABELLED (INCLUDING PATIENT NAME)
- ☐ WHETHER THERE ARE ANY EQUIPMENT PROBLEMS TO BE ADDRESSED
- ☐ SURGEON, ANAESTHESIA PROFESSIONAL AND NURSE REVIEW THE KEY CONCERNS FOR RECOVERY AND MANAGEMENT OF THIS PATIENT

THIS CHECKLIST IS NOT INTENDED TO BE COMPREHENSIVE. ADDITIONS AND MODIFICATIONS TO FIT LOCAL PRACTICE ARE ENCOURAGED.

Figure 1.
World Health Organization- Surgical Safety Checklist (2008).

teamwork and safety climate, suggesting that changes in this attitude may be partially responsible for the effect of the checklist. Also the team's compliance with the checklist is as important as evaluating outcomes.

During the last decades we analyzed the complications occurring in our Spine Surgery Department and reported an overall incidence of complications of 17.3% during three years [14]. Indeed, spinal surgery complications are a relevant and unsolved problem. The incidence of complications in spinal surgery literature ranges between 7% and 20% [15–22].

Nasser et al. [17] performed a systematic evidence-based review of 105 published studies (84 retrospective, 21 prospective) and found a higher incidence of complications (19.9%) in prospective studies compared with retrospective studies (16.1%). The incidence of complications varied widely in spinal surgery literature, even in prospective studies. Rampersaud et al. [23] reported an overall incidence of intraoperative adverse events of 14% (98 adverse events in 700 patients), but only 23 adverse events led to postoperative clinical sequelae. Yadla et al. [16] reported a very high rate of early complications, occurring within 30 days of surgery: global incidence of 53.2%, with a minor complication incidence of 46.4% and a major complication incidence of 21.3%.

It has been also observed that there is no standard definition of complications in spinal surgery literature [23], so it is difficult to compare studies. The Clavien-Dindo and SAVES capture and grading systems [24–26] divide the surgical complications into levels of severity based on the grade of treatment required to face the complication. Glassman et al. classified complications as major or minor: significant complications requiring reoperation or leading to permanent deficit were considered major complications. Other perioperative adverse events with time-limited effect were considered minor complications [27].

To date, few studies have evaluated the effect of complications on clinical outcomes [27–29]. Glassman et al. analyzed a prospective multicenter database for adult spinal deformity to investigate the effects of major and minor complications on disability, pain, postoperative quality of life at 1 year follow up and found that major complications negatively affected the quality of life [27]. However, Fritzell et al. found no significant differences of effects of major and minor complications on 2-years outcomes in three different types of fusion surgery [28]. Grainger et al. examined the relationship between severity of complications and outcomes following Clavien-Dindo classification of complications, and found that the severity of perioperative surgical complications does not appear to influence 1- or 2-years pain and disability outcomes [29]. Lambat et al. performed a large retrospective study and observed that ODI (Oswestry Disability Index) at 2- years follow up was not statistically different between patients having no complications, minor complications or major complications. However, the minimum clinically important difference (MCID) for ODI resulted significantly smaller in the major complication group (31%) than in the minor complication (51%) and no complication groups (65%), demonstrating an impact of complications on the functional outcome [20].

Chen et al. [30] recently performed a 10-week prospective study where SAVES V2 and OrthoSAVES capture systems were used by six orthopedic surgeons and two independent, non-MD clinical reviewers to record adverse events after all elective procedures. They compared the complications rate among groups of patients undergoing spine, hip, knee and shoulder surgery. The first relevant result of this study was the highest rate of complications in spinal surgery compared to the other surgeries; but the most important observation of this study was that overall 99 adverse events were captured by the reviewers, compared with 14 events captured by the surgeons. Surgeons adequately captured major adverse events, but failed to record minor events that were captured by the reviewers; in the spinal surgery group, reviewers captured 45 adverse events versus 8 events captured by surgeons [30].

Considering the high incidence of complications in spinal surgery and their relevant impact for the patients and the health system, during the last years several authors focused their attention on the risk factors related to the onset of complications and on predictive models of complications after spinal surgery [31–35].

Moreover, several preventive measures have been studied and recently described in order to reduce complications in spinal surgery, concerning intraoperative neuromonitoring, blood loss reduction, infections and thrombosis prophylaxis [36–40]. Sethi and co-workers [41] described the application of Lean methodology in spinal surgery. Lean methodology was developed in the manufacturing industry to increase output and decrease costs and then applied in many areas of health care. The authors illustrated a step-by-step process designed specifically to optimize and standardize preoperative, intraoperative and postoperative care for patients undergoing complex spine surgery and they reported a significant reduction of overall complication rate [41].

We proposed to analyze the impact of the introduction of the WHO Surgical Safety Checklist in our Spine Surgery Department, as preventive measure to reduce complications [14].

We retrospectively evaluated the clinical and radiological charts prospectively collected from 917 patients who underwent a spinal surgery procedure from January 2010 to December 2012. The aim of this study was to compare the incidence of complications between two periods, from January to December 2010 (without checklist) and from January 2011 and December 2012 (with checklist) in order to assess the checklist's effectiveness.

We found no correlation between diagnosis and overall complications' incidence. We found a rate of early complications (arising within 1 month after surgery) of 43.3%, a rate of complications requiring surgical revision of 7.6% and a rate of neurological sequelae causing permanent damage of 2.4%. These types of complications have a relevant impact on the health system and, especially the last two categories, on the patients' quality of life and clinical outcomes.

We observed a reduction of the overall incidence of complications following the introduction of the WHO Safety Surgical Checklist: in 2010 without the use of the checklist, the incidence of complications was 24.2%, while in 2011 and 2012 following the checklist introduction, the incidence of complications was 16.7% and 11.7%, respectively (mean 14.2%).

Despite some limitations of our study, the WHO Surgical Safety Checklist resulted to be effective in reducing complications in our Centre.

We recent analyzed also the rate of re-admission and re-operation following spinal surgery. A systematic review [42] of the data concerning the "thirty-day readmission" in spinal surgery indicated percentages between 4.2% and 7.5%, with a variability associated to the presence of one or more centers in which the study takes place and to the type of vertebral pathologies treated. This high frequency is associated with a significant impact from a social and economic point of view, which primarily affects the patient and the National Health System. The most common cause of re-admission was wound complication (39.3%), even if a pooled analysis of risk factors and causes of re-admission was limited by the lack of reporting in spine literature.

Re-admission is very often associated with a re-intervention, or a re-intervention can also occur within the same hospitalization. Our Center treats a wide variety of spinal diseases of oncological, degenerative, traumatic and infectious origin. Therefore we proposed to analyze the rate of re-intervention and surgical revision in the treatment of these pathologies and the causes of these re-operations.

From January 2017 to December 2019, 1260 surgeries were performed at our Spine Surgery Department. Among these, two patients underwent 5 operations, four patients underwent 4 operations, twenty patients underwent 3 operations, 124 patients underwent 2 operations, for a total of 150 patients who underwent more than one spine surgery in a period of three years in the same center (10.7%).

We are now analyzing the causes of these re-operations, which can be a relapse of the disease in the case of oncological pathologies or, for all diagnosis, they can be complications occurring during the follow up period.

A surgical revision is a particularly relevant aspect in assessing the degree of severity of a complication, due to the impact on patient's recovery, and it is relevant also for the economic impact on the National Health System.

We think that a checklist system should be introduced also during the pre-operative and post-operative phases, in order to highlight all the key steps where complications can arise, not only during surgery. The introduction and validation of these checklists, implemented for pre-operative, intra-operative and post-operative phases, should be followed by the identification of targeted actions to prevent complications, improve patients' safety and reduce the economic impact.

Following the WHO Surgical Safety Checklist, a checklist for the complex process of ward round (WR) was developed by Caldwell et al. in 2011 [43] and it has been recently implemented and evaluated through different studies. The prime objective of ward round is to assess the clinical state of the inpatient and plan further management. For WR assessment it is fundamental the gathering of new information and reviewing of information already available. Additional information are provided by verbal communication with the patient and the family, nursing staff, medical colleagues, patient examination, clinical charts, pathology and radiological investigations. Such assessment allows a rational approach to further management including the alteration of therapy, arranging further investigations or surgery, referral to other specialists, planning the discharge. In a busy surgical ward round there is the potential to overlook important aspects of care, their documentation and communication. So the use of a checklist during medical ward round has been described by Caldwell [43] with consideration of key aspects of care being bedside consultation, patient safety, chart review, planning and appropriate documentation. Pitcher et al. [44] implemented and evaluated the WR checklist: they identified the deficiencies in general surgical WRs and the benefits of a checklist approach in overcoming this. Initially, members of the surgical team were unaware of the checklist and some deficiencies were detected. Subsequently, the team was prompted against the checklist and during the ward rounds a designated member of the team acted as 'prompter' if aspects of care were not considered according to the checklist. A structured ward round progress form was developed and it was assessed before and after specific education in its use. This form was based on the original checklist and became an integral part of the medical record. Following the use of the checklist and prompting during ward rounds, a significant improvement occurred for the majority of criteria included in the checklist, all of which reached statistical significance. The introduction of the structured progress form, even with prompting, did not initially improve documentation but this was substantially improved with specific education. The authors concluded that the use of a checklist during surgical ward rounds improved consideration of most key aspects of care and education in the completion of a structured progress form substantially improved documentation. A randomized controlled trial of the impact of surgical WR checklist conducted in a simulated environment showed improved standardization, evidence-based management of post-operative complications and quality of ward round [45].

A WR checklist was introduced also on orthopedic ward round and evaluated by a prospective cohort study [46]. The authors observed that after introduction of the checklist, daily documentation of surgical details improved from 38.6% to 85.3%

of patient encounters. Fasting status documentation improved from 9.1% to 70.6% of patient encounters. Venous thromboembolism prophylaxis documentation increased from 6.8% to 92.6%. Documentation of weight-bearing status improved from 11.4% to 83.8%. Thus, the use of a structured checklist during orthopedic ward rounds led to significant improvement in both the consideration and the documentation of key aspects of surgical care.

These findings were recently confirmed by Krishnamohan and co-workers [47] who implemented and assessed a surgical WR checklist for daily surgical ward rounds. The authors observed that the overall documentation of the six parameters analyzed improved following implementation of the WR checklist (from 26% pre-checklist to 79% post-checklist). In particular, documentation of assessment of fluid balance improved from 8–76%. The key parameters analyzed were: VTE prescribed, Antibiotics reviewed, Fluid balance reviewed, Blood tests reviewed, Patient observations, Drug chart. These selected parameters were identified as often overlooked or inadequately reviewed during surgical WR. The checklist helped bring focus to these aspects of care and the number of adverse events reported decreased following WR checklist implementation. Subsequent audit at 3 months post-checklist implementation maintained improvement with documentation at 72%. The authors concluded that the WR checklist benefits patient safety. It improves communication, documentation and ensure that key issues are not missed at patient assessment on WRs.

3. Conclusions

The data reported underline the relevance of checklist systems to improve patients' safety and clinical outcomes. Effects on morbidity and mortality after introduction of safety checklists have been investigated in several studies [10, 48–51]. Systematic reviews find evidence in favor of checklist use having effects on patient outcomes such as reduced complications [10, 49, 50], wound infections [50] blood loss [50] and mortality rates [49, 50]. Checklist use suggested improved outcomes in high-risk pediatric surgery in developing countries [51].

Their use also contributes to improved information transfer and communication in different phases of surgery [52]. Very few studies report any negative patient outcome effects when using checklists [53], but implementation requires time and effort [2] because a "culture of safety" is required. Still, some studies report no reduction of complications or mortality [54, 55]. A more recent publication reported a lowered mortality rate but no changes in complication rates [56]. Russ et al. [57] observed that the quality of operating room teamwork and communication was improved due to more sharing of case critical information, better decision-making and team coordination, openness about knowledge gaps, and improved team cohesion. In a climate of greater safety for the patient and improved outcome, the use of checklists should influence the operating room (or ward round) work processes so as to have an impact on patient outcome and in this context the teamwork is crucial.

During the last decade, teamwork has been addressed as interprofessional practice or collaboration and described by attributes of this practice such as: interdependence of professional actions, focus on user needs, negotiation between professionals, shared decision making, mutual respect and trust among professionals, and acknowledgment of the role and work of the different professional groups. Teamwork and interprofessional collaboration are considered as a strategy for effective organization of health care services because the complexity of healthcare requires integration of knowledge and practices from different professional groups.

Health organizations in western countries are committed to improving patient safety through education of staff and teamwork education programs, including the use of checklists and other tools dedicated to improving clinical outcomes.

Acknowledgements

The authors thank Carlo Piovani for his helpful collaboration.

Funding

The research was partially funded by the grant "Ricerca Finalizzata 2016" from the Italian Ministry of Health.

Conflict of interest

The authors declare no conflict of interest.

Author details

Giovanni Barbanti Brodano[1], Cristiana Griffoni[1*], Alessandro Ricci[2], Sandra Giannone[2], Daniela Francesca Ghisi[2] and Alessandro Gasbarrini[1]

1 Department of Oncological and Degenerative Spine Surgery, IRCCS Istituto Ortopedico Rizzoli, Bologna, Italy

2 Department of Anesthesia and Intensive Care, IRCCS Istituto Ortopedico Rizzoli, Bologna, Italy

*Address all correspondence to: cristiana.griffoni@ior.it

IntechOpen

© 2020 The Author(s). Licensee IntechOpen. This chapter is distributed under the terms of the Creative Commons Attribution License (http://creativecommons.org/licenses/by/3.0), which permits unrestricted use, distribution, and reproduction in any medium, provided the original work is properly cited.

References

[1] Weiser TG, Regenbogen SE, Thompson KD, Haynes AB, Lipsitz SR, Berry WR, et al. An estimation of the global volume of surgery: A modelling strategy based on available data. Lancet. 2008;**372**:139-144

[2] deVries EN, Ramrattan MA, Smorenburg SM, Gouma DJ, Boermeester MA. The incidence and nature of in-hospital adverse events: A systematic review. Quality & Safety in Health Care. 2008;**17**:216-223

[3] McCoy CC, Englum BR, Keenan JE, Vaslef SN, Shapiro ML, Scarborough JE. Impact of specific postoperative complications on the outcomes of emergency general surgery patients. Journal of Trauma and Acute Care Surgery. 2015;**78**:912-919

[4] Storesund A, Haugen AS, Hjortas M, Nortvedt MW, Flaaten H, Eide GE, et al. Accuracy of surgical complication rate estimation using ICD-10 codes. The British Journal of Surgery. 2019;**106**:236-244

[5] Weerakkody RA, Cheshire NJ, Riga C, Lear R, Hamady MS, Moorthy K, et al. Surgical technology and operating room safety failure: A systematic review of quantitative studies. BMJ Quality and Safety. 2013;**22**:710-718

[6] Provonost P, Needdham D, Berenholtz S, Sinopoli D, Chu H, Cosgrove S, et al. An intervention to decrease catheter- related bloodstream infections in the ICU. N Engl Med. 2006;**355**:2725-2731

[7] Dixon-Woods M, Leslie M, Tarrant C, Bion J. Explaining matching Michigan: An ethnographic study of a patient safety program. Implementation Science. 2013;**8**:70

[8] Haynes AB, Weiser TG, Berry WR, Lipsitz SR, Breizat AH, Dellinger EP, et al. Safe surgery saves lives study group: A surgical safety checklist to reduce morbidity and mortality in a global population. N Engl Med. 2009;**360**:491-499

[9] Weiser TG, Haynes AB, Lashoher A, Dziekan G, Boorman DJ, Berry WR, et al. Perspectives in quality: Designing the WHO surgical safety Chacklist. International Journal for Quality in Health Care. 2010;**22**:365-370

[10] Bergs J, Hellings J, Cleemput I, Zurel Ö, De Troyer V, Van Hiel M, et al. Systematic review and meta-analysis of the effect of the World Health Organization surgical safety checklist on postoperative complications. The British Journal of Surgery. 2014;**101**:150-158

[11] Haugen AS, Softeland E, Almeland SK, et al. Effect of the World Health Organization checklist on patient outcomes: A stepped wedge cluster randomized controlled trial. Annals of Surgery. 2015;**261**:821-828

[12] Lepänluoma M, Rahi M, Takala R, Loyttyniemi E, Ikonen TS. Analysis of neurosurgical reoperations: Use of a surgical checklist and reduction of infection-related and preventable complication-related reoperations. Journal of Neurosurgery. 2015;**123**:145-152

[13] Haynes AB, Weiser TG, Berry WR, Lipsitz SR, Breizat A-HS, Dellinger EP, et al. Changes in safety attitude and relationship to decreased postoperative morbidity and mortality following implementation of a checklist-based surgical safety intervention. BMJ Quality and Safety. 2011;**20**:102-107

[14] Barbanti Brodano G, Griffoni C, Halme J, Tedesco G, Terzi S, Bandiera S, et al. Spinal surgery complications: An unsolved problem- is the World Health Organization safety surgical checklist

an useful tool to reduce them? European Spine Journal. 2019 Nov 6. DOI: 10.1007/s00586-019-06203-x

[15] Ratliff JK, Lebude B, Albert T, Anene-Maidoh T, Anderson G, Dagostino P, et al. Complications in spinal surgery: Comparative survey of spine surgeons and patients who underwent spinal surgery. Journal of Neurosurgery. Spine. 2009;**10**:578-584

[16] Yadla S, Malone J, Campbell PG, Maltenfort MG, Harrop JS, Sharan AD, et al. Early complications in spine surgery and relation to preoperative diagnosis: A single-center prospective study. Journal of Neurosurgery. Spine. 2010;**13**:360-366

[17] Nasser R, Yadla S, Maltenfort MG, Harrop JS, Anderson DG, Vaccaro AR, et al. Complications in spine surgery. A review. J Neurosurg Spine. 2010;**13**:144-157

[18] Deyo RA, Cherkin DC, Loeser JD, Bigos SJ, Ciol MA. Morbidity and mortality in association with operations on the lumbar spine. The influence of age, diagnosis, and procedure. The Journal of Bone and Joint Surgery. American Volume. 1992;**74**:536-543

[19] Patil CG, Lad SP, Santarelli J, Boakye M. National inpatient complications and outcomes after surgery for spinal metastasis from 1993-2002. Cancer. 2007;**110**:625-630

[20] Lambat MP, Glassman SD, Carreon LY. Impact of perioperative complications on clinical outcome scores in lumbar fusion surgery. Journal of Neurosurgery. Spine. 2013;**18**:265-268

[21] Fu KM, Smith JS, Polly DW, et al. Morbidity and mortality in the surgical treatment of 10,329 adults with degenerative lumbar stenosis. Journal of Neurosurgery. Spine. 2010;**12**:443-446

[22] Campbell PG, Yadla S, Malone J, Maltenfort MG, Harrop JS, Sharan AD, et al. Complications related to instrumentation in spine surgery: A prospective analysis. Neurosurgical Focus. 2011;**31**:E10

[23] Rampersaud YR, Moro ER, Neary MA, White K, Lewis SJ, Massicotte EM, et al. Intraoperative adverse events and related postoperative complications in spine surgery: Implications for enhancing patient safety founded on evidence-based protocols. Spine (Phila Pa 1976). 2006;**31**:1503-1510

[24] Dindo D, Demartines N, Clavien PA. Classification of surgical complications: A new proposal with evaluation in a cohort of 6336 patients and results of a survey. Annals of Surgery. 2004;**240**:205-213

[25] Rampersaud YR, Neary MA, White K. Spine adverse events severity system: Content validation and interobserver reliability assessment. Spine (Phila Pa 1976). 2010;**35**:790-795

[26] Rampersaud YR, Anderson PA, Dimar JR 2nd, Fisher CG, Spine Trauma Study Group and Degenerative Spine Study Group. Spinal adverse events severity system, version 2 (SAVES-V2): Inter- and intraobserver reliability assessment. Journal of Neurosurgery. Spine. 2016;**25**:256-263

[27] Glassman SD, Hamill CL, Bridwell KH, Schwab FJ, Dimar JR, Lowe TG. The impact of perioperative complications on clinical outcome in adult deformity surgery. Spine (Phila Pa 1976). 2007;**32**:2764-2770

[28] Fritzell P, Hägg O, Nordwall A. Complications in lumbar fusion surgery for chronic low back pain: Comparison of three surgical techniques used in a prospective randomized study. A report from the Swedish lumbar spine study group. European Spine Journal. 2003;**12**:178-189

[29] Grainger J, Hammett T, Isaacs R, Cook C. Influence of perioperative complication severity on 1- and 2-year outcomes of low back surgery. Journal of Orthopaedics and Traumatology. 2017;**18**:127-134

[30] Chen BP, Garland K, Roffey DM, Poitras S, Dervin G, Lapner P, et al. Can surgeons adequately capture adverse events using the spinal adverse events severity system (SAVES) and OrthoSAVES? Clinical Orthopaedics and Related Research. 2017;**475**:253-260

[31] Molina CS, Thakore RV, Blumer A, Obremskey WT, Sethi MK. Use of the National Surgical Quality Improvement Program in orthopaedic surgery. Clinical Orthopaedics and Related Research. 2015;**473**:1574-1581

[32] Sugrue PA, Halpin RJ, Koski TR. Treatment algorithms and protocol practice in high-risk spine surgery. Neurosurgery Clinics of North America. 2013;**24**:219-230

[33] Bekelis K, Desai A, Bakhoum SF, Missios S. A predictive model of complications after spine surgery: The National Surgical Quality Improvement Program (NSQIP) 2005-2010. The Spine Journal. 2014;**14**:1247-1255

[34] Lee MJ, Hacquebord J, Varshney A, Cizik AM, Bransford RJ, Bellabarba C, et al. Risk factors for medical complication after lumbar spine surgery: A multivariate analysis of 767 patients. Spine (Phila Pa 1976). 2011;**36**:1801-1806

[35] Lee MJ, Cizik AM, Hamilton D, Chapman JR. Predicting medical complications after spine surgery: A validated model using a prospective surgical registry. The Spine Journal. 2014;**14**:291-299

[36] Belykh E, Carotenuto A, Kalinin AA, Akshulakov SK, Kerimbayev T, Borisov VE, et al. Surgical Protocol for Infections, Nonhealing Wound Prophylaxis, and Analgesia: Development and Implementation for Posterior Spinal Fusions. World Neurosurg. 2019;**123**:390-401.e2

[37] Mosenthal WP, Landy DC, Boyajian HH, Idowu OA, Shi LL, Ramos E, et al. Thromboprophylaxis in spinal surgery. Spine (Phila Pa 1976). 2018;**43**:E474-E481

[38] Daniel JW, Botelho RV, Milano JB, Dantas FR, Onishi FJ, Neto ER, et al. Intraoperative neurophysiological monitoring in spine surgery: A systematic review and meta-analysis. Spine (Phila Pa 1976). 2018;**43**:1154-1160

[39] Lu VM, Ho YT, Nambiar M, Mobbs RJ, Phan K. The perioperative efficacy and safety of antifibrinolytics in adult spinal fusion surgery: A systematic review and meta-analysis. Spine (Phila Pa 1976). 2018;**43**:E949-E958

[40] Ali ZS, Ma TS, Ozturk AK, Malhotra NR, Schuster JM, Marcotte PJ, et al. Pre-optimization of spinal surgery patients: Development of a neurosurgical enhanced recovery after surgery (ERAS) protocol. Clinical Neurology and Neurosurgery. 2018;**164**:142-153

[41] Sethi R, Yanamadala V, Burton DC, Bess RS. Using lean process improvement to enhance safety and value in orthopaedic surgery: The case of spine surgery. The Journal of the American Academy of Orthopaedic Surgeons. 2017;**25**:e244-e250

[42] Bernatz JT, Anderson PA. Thirty-day readmission rates in spine surgery: systematic review and meta-analysis. Neurosurgical Focus. 2015;**39**(4):E7

[43] Herring R, Desai T, Caldwell G. Quality and safety at the point of care: How long should a ward round take? Clinical Medicine. 2011;**11**:20-22

[44] Pitcher M, Lin JTW, Thompson G, Tayaran A, Chan S. Implementation and evaluation of a checklist to improve patient care on surgical WRs. ANZ Journal of Surgery. 2016;**86**:356-360

[45] Pucher PH, Aggarwal R, Qurashi M, Singh P, Darzi A. Randomized clinical trial of the impact of surgical ward-care checklists on postoperative care in a simulated environment. The British Journal of Surgery. 2014;**101**:1666-1673

[46] Talia AJ, Drummond J, Muirhead C, Tran P. Using a structured checklist to improve the orthopedic ward round: A prospective cohort study. Orthopedics. 2017;**40**:e663-e667

[47] Krishnamohan N, Maitra I, Shetty VD. The surgical ward checklist: Improving patient safety and clinical documentation. Journal of Multidisciplinary Healthcare. 2019;**12**:789-794

[48] Treadwell JR, Lucas S, Tsou AY. Surgical checklists: A systematic review of impacts and implementation. BMJ Quality and Safety. 2014;**23**:299-318

[49] Borchard A, Schwappach DL, Barbir A, Bezzola P. A systematic review of the effectiveness, compliance, and critical factors for implementation of safety checklists in surgery. Annals of Surgery. 2012;**256**:925-933

[50] Gillespie BM, Chaboyer W, Thalib L, John M, Fairweather N, Slater K. Effect of using a safety checklist on patient complications after surgery: A systematic review and meta-analysis. Anesthesiology. 2014;**120**:1380-1389

[51] Lagoo J, Lopushinsky SR, Haynes AB, Bain P, Flageole H, Skarsgard ED, et al. Effectiveness and meaningful use of paediatric surgical safety checklists and their implementation strategies: A systematic review with narrative synthesis. BMJ Open. 2017;7:1-13

[52] Nagpal K, Vats A, Lamb B, Ashrafian H, Sevdalis N, Vincent C, et al. Information transfer and communication in surgery: A systematic review. Annals of Surgery. 2010;**252**:225-239

[53] Thomassen Ø, Storesund A, Søfteland E, Brattebø G. The effects of safety checklists in medicine: A systematic review. Acta Anaesthesiologica Scandinavica. 2014;**58**:5-18

[54] Urbach DR, Govindarajan A, Saskin R, Wilton AS, Baxter NN. Introduction of surgical safety checklists in Ontario, Canada. The New England Journal of Medicine. 2014;**370**:1029-1038

[55] Lübbeke A, Hovaguimian F, Wickboldt N, Barea C, Clergue F, Hoffmeyer P, et al. Effectiveness of the surgical safety checklist in a high standard care environment. Medical Care. 2013;**51**:425-429

[56] Abbott TEF, Ahmad T, Phull MK, Fowler AJ, Hewson R, Biccard BM, et al. The surgical safety checklist and patient outcomes after surgery: A prospective observational cohort study, systematic review and meta-analysis. British Journal of Anaesthesia. 2018;**120**:146-155

[57] Russ S, Rout S, Sevdalis N, Moorthy K, Darzi A, Vincent C. Do safety checklists improve teamwork and communication in the operating room?: A systematic review. Annals of Surgery. 2013;**258**:856-871

Chapter 7

Learning from Errors

Gabor Xantus and Laszlo Zavori

Abstract

The authors of this chapter have worked in emergency care in 5 countries on 4 continents in the past 9 years. In their experience, acute care anywhere in the world shares two main features; strong teamwork and tremendous mental, physical, and psychological stress. The significant workload, both on individual and team levels, render the care system vulnerable to human errors, which can unfortunately be detrimental to patients and staff alike. Due to the commonalities it is not surprising that health care professionals tend to make similar mistakes irrespective of economic, cultural, religious aspect or healthcare settings. We opine that mistakes are not necessarily and exclusively bad things, but invaluable opportunities for improvement. In this chapter, the authors aim to introduce the concept of learning from errors to the readers. Numerous studies and books have already been published on the subject, so anyone could rightfully ask, why read another study? The answer is straightforward, unlike other articles, this chapter invites the reader to work together with the authors through a real-world case. The text will guide the reader through the topic painlessly in a step-by-step fashion offering plenty of opportunity to practice and reflect on the newly acquired knowledge. Global healthcare is facing significant changes these days. Learning from errors may be the initial step to help move away from the blame and shame culture and build a new system which should be based on solid partnership and respect between patients and carers. Such a new, supportive and compassionate system could provide higher quality care and at the same time, protect practitioners from burnout and stress ensuring that healthcare jobs are not only work but a life-long fulfilling career.

Keywords: human factors, human error, adverse event, risk assessment, root cause analysis, feedback loop

1. Introduction

What is human error and how can we learn from them?

According to UK hospital literature data, at least one in ten patients is certain to suffer some level of harm during their care [1]. If true, it is a terrifying proposition, resulting in about 600,000 incidents per year in Great Britain alone. This is in comparison to the aviation industry, where fatalities have never exceeded 0.6 cases per million flights (14 deaths) [Civil Aviation Authority]. In the aviation sector, each incident must be investigated by law, however, there are no similar legal obligations for health care providers despite the significantly higher numbers of incidents and fatalities.

How can we improve healthcare related harm? Shall we introduce additional protocols and checklists similar to practice ibn the aviation sector? Does each complaint or error need a thorough analysis to better understand what could have led to the incident at both individual and organisational level? Is this data applicable to different health care systems or UK specific? If this proportion of harm is not country specific, how can we learn from each other?

The authors opine that there is no single good answer, but rather a series of answers, which together can help to understand and solve the problem of accidental, preventable harm in healthcare. In this chapter, we present a real-life incident and aim to guide the reader to implement both an industrial and a health care related algorithm to recognise, analyse and synthesise the learning points of the exemplary error. We also would like to spark further discussions and invite any interested readers to a best practice sharing session at the end of the chapter. We encourage everybody to join/start any blog in this topic to spread the word about the importance of learning from errors in health care.

The fast pace of modern medicine is mostly driven by patient's demand for a quick fix, however this tempo does not result in a faultless operation. The often-unreasonable hurry is likely one of the reasons why the emergency speciality has unfortunately claimed a silver medallist position on the podium of litigation, not far behind the surgical disciplines [2, 3]. Clearly, other factors, like the immense stress, the constant pressure to make back-to-back decisions and perform various procedures under severe time pressure are also inherently incident prone. Speed comes at a price that is mostly paid by the patient but often the health care provider as well (second victim). The other element that attracts mistakes is the number of interruptions during the process of care. A typical patient journey in the emergency department includes countless stops, each with a brief handover between providers of different qualifications (ambulance, triage nurse, doctor, etc.). Handovers are knowingly dangerous in medicine. Everyone knows the Chinese whisper when a sentence conveyed ear-to-ear in a line of people. By the time the message reaches the end, the original text is barely recognisable. Unsurprisingly, according to regulatory bodies, one of the most common errors in emergency departments is loss of data [4, 5].

Human errors are events when a planned action fails to achieve the desired result due to a human failure. In this chapter we introduce both an ergonomic based industrial approach and hospital protocols used in the UK. Both methods are excellent not only for recognising an error or even a near miss. They are also useful at mitigating consequential damage, mapping the factors leading to the incident, and also preventing possible future occurrences and instigating the necessary corrective measures (**Figure 1**). The explicit goal of the ergonomic approach is the optimization of equipment design and reduction of work-related stress to minimise chances of human errors (International Civil Aviation Organisation). Even though similar initiatives are seen in medicine, as of yet there is no overarching authority to enforce necessary measures.

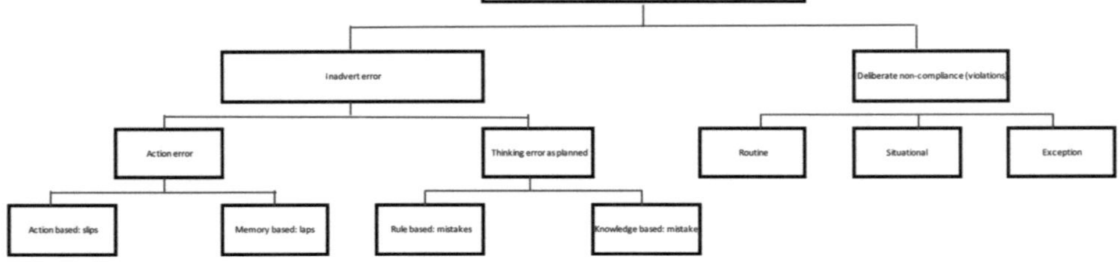

Figure 1.
Ergonomic flowchart for processing human omission categories.

1.1 Adverse event recognition

In the UK, Australia, Canada and the USA, dedicated systems are in place to facilitate incident recognition and reporting. Most enable users to anonymously (or named) report any adverse occurrence. The systems are designed to alert manager levels and prompt actions according to pre-set protocols.

In the next paragraphs, we present an incident from a real ED (**Box 1** and **2**). The reader will be asked to review the incident and use their experience to work up the error as normal (according to local protocols/experience). An ergonomic flow chart will then be shown and the reader should compare the two approaches and mark their thoughts in the below workbook.

Incident Log entry: A patient complained to a senior nurse on the Clinical Decision Unit of the Emergency Department during a busy shift. The nurse made an entry to the incident log saying: *"a patient complained that the senior doctor referred her to Mental Health Services without consulting her"*.

Box 1.
The summary of the clinical incident.

Workbook 1.

Result of the usual approach:
Result of the ergonomic approach:
Result of the repeated ergonomic assessment:

Broader context (for those unfamiliar with UK Mental Health protocols)
The Mental Capacity Act (MCA) was designed to protect and empower people who may lack the mental capacity to make their own decisions about their care and treatment. It applies to people aged 16 and over. The MCA refers to decisions about day-to-day situations and giving consent to medical interventions including surgery. There are 5 principles of the MCA and all practitioners must act in the best interest of the patients and presume that anybody under their care has the capacity to make a decision themselves, unless it's proved otherwise. Furthermore, any health care worker must make sure to help people make their own decisions, whenever it is feasible.
In this case, despite the registrar believing to have acted in the best interest of the patient, he breached the protocols by not discussing his working diagnosis of potential postpartum depression and the steps he deemed necessary to help the patient. As the MCA states people must be encouraged "to express their preferences for care and treatment" the registrar should have discussed all available options detailing the presumed benefit and exploring the patient's understanding of the help offered. In addition, the registrar should have assessed potential cultural barriers, as in some cases, depression (or any mental health diagnosis) might be seen stigmatising and shameful.

In incident management, sometimes multiple answers are available for the same question. To give the benefit of doubt, the reader is asked to repeat the ergonomic exercise using the other arm of the process. If, during the above, the reader responded that the error was "Intentional Non-Compliance" (i.e., the junior doctor knowingly violated departmental regulations by failing to record vital parameters, to seek senior advice before transferring the patient and did not hand over the patient to the nurse in charge of the clinical decision unit) they should consider choosing the alternative path of "Inadvertent error/incomplete knowledge" (the junior was not aware of the regular transfer process and/or undervalued the patient's condition). One must realise that both solutions (and even a combination of the two) are equally conceivable however, each involves different corrective steps.

> **Example 1.** The patient attended two consecutive days with back pain. She was post-partum (3 weeks) and was alone with her first baby. During her previous attendances she was sent home with analgesia and referral to physio. Last night was admitted for "rest and review" as she claimed that the pain killers were ineffective. In the morning ward round, the patient was seen by a locum registrar, who suspected social isolation (husband was abroad and there was no family support for the patient) and potential post-partum depression. The registrar ran his clinical judgement by the consultant in charge who agreed on referral to social/psychological support. The registrar called social services and was informed by a secretary that post-partum patients are seen by the Crisis Team. The secretary recorded the patient details and promised the registrar that someone will call him back from her team. After the referral was made the registrar tended to his further duties on the Clinical Decision Unit (CDU).
>
> The incident log entry said: "*a patient complained that the senior doctor referred her to Mental Health Services without consulting with her*".
>
> **Question 1: What type of error do you anticipate?**
>
> - Poor handover.
> - Records not available.
> - Documentation/Tracking issue.

Box 2.
The full extent of the incident.

1.2 Background events and risk analysis

Once an incident was recognised, the immediate harm was mitigated the background and context needs further assessment. Again, the health care approach is different to the ergonomic one. Without a detailed understanding of the circumstances and background facts, causes cannot be fully determined. Without fully exploring the causes, potential future recurrence of similar incidents cannot be prevented. Therefore, it is in the best interest of any system to learn the crucial details.

The reader shall review the below two charts (**Figure 2**; **Table 1**) and mark their ideas on risk assessment in Workbook 2.

Workbook 2.

Ideas generated by the ergonomic approach
Ideas generated by the healthcare approach

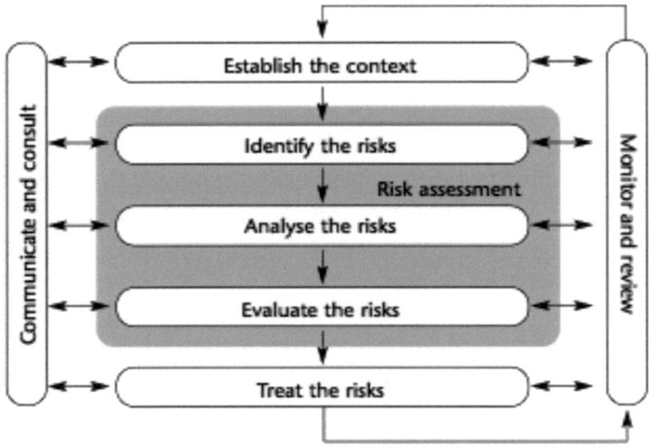

Figure 2.
Ergonomic flow chart for risk assessment.

Likelihood score	Rare	Unlikely	Possible	Likely	Almost certain
	Will probably never happen/ recur	Unlikely to happen again/ recur, but it may do so	Might happen or recur occasionally	Will probably happen/recur but it is not a pressing issue	Will surey happen/recur possibly frequently
Catastrophic	5	10	15	20	25
Major	4	8	12	16	20
Moderate	3	6	9	12	15
Minor	2	4	6	8	10
Negligible	1	2	3	4	5

Low risk = 1–3; Moderate risk = 4–6, High risk = 8–12; Extreme risk = 15–25.

Table 1.
Incident likelihood and risk scoring (risk scoring = consequence x likelihood).

1.3 Investigating the causes

The UK hospital practice has currently advocated three methods to identify causation: the formal "Root Cause Analysis" (RCA), the "fishbone" approach, and the "5 - why" (5 W) method. There are no set rules as to when to implement a certain method, however, a rule of thumb is that an RCA is used to analyse complex, severe, and/or frequently recurring problems, while the "fishbone," or 5 W method, is reserved for simpler incidents [6–8].

As in our present example, the patient did not suffer permanent health impairment and the number of involved of staff was less than 5 people. The 5 W method was used in the investigation process. The advantages of this approach are that it does not take a long time but creates an opportunity for a layered analysis. The technique is simple; the investigator should ask a minimum of 5 questions starting with "Why". If the problem cannot be explored in depth even after the 5th question then either, additional questions can be raised or a new method is needed to investigate further. The disadvantage of the 5 W method is its subjectivity: no matter how unbiased the investigator, their cultural, cognitive, and emotional factors can affect the result. To address this source bias (if resources allow), two independent investigators are advised to be put on the case. Given the length of the article, the fishbone and RCA approach cannot be presented at this time, however, the reader is encouraged to review these methods based on the references provided.

The reader is asked to formulate their own 5 questions and enter in the workbook. Once finished, please review the questions raised by the hospital investigator (see **Table 2**). Compare the questions and make notes of the differences. What does the difference suggest to the reader?

Table 2 Summary of the given clinical incident according to the 5 W method.

Workbook 3.

Question 1.
Question 2.
Question 3.
Question 4.
Question 5.

The differences between the readers and the investigators questions:
1. **Why** was the patient admitted to CDU last night?
2. **Why** was her social circumstances and mental health status not assessed during prior visits?
3. **Why** did the registrar forget to tell the patient his suspicion of a potential post-partum depression?
4. **Why** did Crisis Team not call back the registrar?
5. **Why** did the registrar check back at the patient?
Please reflect on the differences

Question	Answer
Why was the patient admitted to CDU last night?	As the patient presented with the same complaints twice (unplanned return), per department policy she should have been seen by a consultant. The night shift was very busy, the consultant on call was unavailable, therefore the night registrar admitted the patient to the CDU.
Why was her social circumstances and mental health status not assessed during prior visits?	The patient was seen by two different juniors and the case was discussed with two different seniors. There was no mention of the social or mental health assessment as the juniors did not think about it.
Why did the registrar forget to tell the patient his suspicion of a potential post-partum depression?	The registrar was very busy with other patients and thought that once spoken to by someone from the Crisis Team he will discharge the patient with a home appointment with a counsellor.
Why did Crisis Team not call back the registrar?	The Crisis Team assessed another patient at the medical ward and thought to that they would quickly see the patient.
Why did the registrar check back at the patient?	The patient was seen by the Crisis. Team and as she refused any further intervention (she felt offended by the stigmatising label of depression) the CDU charge nurse offered her a self-discharge form. By the time the registrar returned to review, the patient had left.

Table 2.
Summary of the investigators "5-whys" of the above error.

1.4 Significance of the adverse events

The previous paragraphs helped the reader to review a real-world, potentially dangerous incident, identify the involved parties, have a detailed background check, categorise the error leading to the incident, perform a quick risk assessment, and address immediate threats. In the next section, we will determine the learning points and decide who shall learn to prevent further occurrences.

This is a key step in the process, as the severity of any particular incident is determined by the weight of the consequences and the frequency of potential reoccurrence. These evaluation steps will also reveal the nature of necessary corrective actions on both an individual and organisational level. In Anglo-Saxon areas, health care institutions use a very similar nomenclature/protocols for reporting incidents: minor events ("near miss", "quasi-damage", or "minimal damage") should only be reported to the immediate supervisor (as is practical, but preferably within 12 hours), whose task it is to investigate, resolve or take it forward. However, moderate/severe incidents should be reported immediately not only to the line manager, but the director in charge. In most cases, the reporting system automatically notifies the appropriate level. "Serious" or "catastrophic" events should be immediately taken to the hospital directorship level. The reader is asked to review

Likelihood score	**Rare**	**Unlikely**	**Possible**	**Likely**	**Almost certain**
	Will probably never happen/ recur	Unlikely to happen again/ recur, but it may do so	Might happen or recur occasionally	Will probably happen/recur but it is not a pressing issue	Will surey happen/recur possibly frequently
Catastrophic	5	10	15	20	25
Major	4	8	12	16	20
Moderate	3	6	9	12	15
Minor	2	4	6	8	10
Negligible	1	2	3	4	5

Low risk = 1-3; Moderate risk = 4-6, High risk = 8-12; Extreme risk = 15-25.

Table 3.
Incident likelihood and risk scoring (risk scoring = consequence x likelihood).

Table 3, which summarises the categories used by a UK tertiary hospital. In the workbook please enter the differences between the reader's system and the UK system to reflect on the advantages/disadvantages of both.

Workbook 4.

Summary of the reader's local system
Reflection on differences between the UK and the reader's own system (if applicable)

1.5 Closing the loop, feedback to the team

Identifying and classifying adverse events, analysing the relevant risks, determining the likelihood of recurrence and determining lessons at both individual and organisational level is pointless without communicating the result to the individuals involved and (while maintaining anonymity) with the entire team. If this step is missed, the opportunity to learn from error will be lost forever, not to mention that the incident will surely reoccur [9].

In the author's experience, the UK is at the forefront of recognising, managing and learning from errors and incidents with a nearly two decade-long history in the NHS. The National Quality Committee issued a document in 2013 (Concordat 2013) promoting the culture of learning from errors, the importance of timely feedback and the culture of candour. While the concordat is mostly a manifesto, another national organisation, the National Reporting and Learning Service, developed a seven-step tool to help with the practical application of this relatively new concept into the day-to-day operation.

However, even the English system has minor flaws. NHS England does not have a uniform reporting system and procedure, rather, it is left to hospitals to choose the best method. Most Trusts have their own classification system, which may differ significantly from one another. Unfortunately, these differences can conceal system-wide problems, so many advocate the need in favour of a unified, national system. Inarguably, a single system, similar to aviation, would simplify detection, facilitate detection and management of adverse events, as well as provide all level healthcare staff with transferable skills that can be applied in practice and used anywhere in the country.

Using **Table 4** as a guide the reader should review the example of a clinical error and mark their recommendation in the workbook. Once the exercise is complete please review their answers against the hospital investigator's recommendations (**Table 5**) and reflect on the differences.

Workbook 5.

The reader's recommendations
Reflection on the differences

1.6 Barriers to learning from errors?

In the final section of the chapter we will have a quick trouble-shooting run-through to identify the potential barriers. At the moment, in the Anglo-Saxon territories incident recognition is based on voluntary reporting hence can only be as effective as often it is used.

The first difficulty stems from the inherent weakness of any self-reporting voluntary system; any non-mandatory, non-punitive, but at the same time non-incentivising activity depends solely on the level of motivation of those carrying out the activity. Not surprisingly, the sensitivity of hospital incident reporting systems (i.e. how many events does the system detect at all) is around 30% [10], while its specificity (i.e. how the detection rate relates to actual errors) is even lower: 14% [11].

To explain the poor sensitivity and specificity, similar answers were found throughout the world, regardless of political setting, religion, culture, or even

NRLS steps
Build a safety culture
Lead and support your staff
Integrate your risk management activity
Promote reporting
Involve and communicate with patients and the public
Learn and share safety lessons
Implement solutions to prevent harm

Table 4.
Summary of the NRLS 7 steps.

Trust measures to mitigate errors
No patient can self-discharge with an alleged mental health issue.
Patients with alleged mental health issues needs senior review prior discharge.
CDU Lead to revise CDU review policies and Mental Health Referral pathway.
Promote and appraise reporting.
Duty of Candour applies, patient shall be called and a formal letter might be considered.
Learning points to be discussed on nursing training day and junior teaching.
Compulsory CDU checklist prior to (self) discharge.

Table 5.
The investigators recommendation based on the above NRLS tool.

clinical setting, whether inpatient and outpatient care, hospital or GP practice. This similarity highlights the importance of the human factors in reporting. A USA primary care survey found [12] that the time spent writing a report was inversely proportional to the frequency of reporting. Iranian authors [13] found that hospital workers reported only half of serious medication errors. According to their results, fears of accusations, retaliation, and the reporting burden ("it takes too long to write") were the main disincentives behind non-reporting. It was also clear from the responses that almost all practitioners stated in unison that "there is no need to report if there was no problem with the patient". The barriers of reporting seem to be similar in Canada: according to a hospital study [14], the timing of the reports was proportionate with factors perceived important by the responders: incidents endangering patient or staff safety, while the time spent writing the report, or the user unfriendly reporting interface significantly slowed down reporting speed. According to the study, professional identity, lack of information, unclear organisational relationships, and fear of retaliation also proved to be important barriers. Another Iranian article [15] concluded that the main barriers to reporting were the lack of effective reporting systems, complicated forms and the lack of collegial support. They also concurred with other studies that incidents perceived as minor were less frequently reported. The study highlighted significant differences between genders and occupations: women tend to report earlier than men, and nursing staff are more likely to report in writing than doctors. Most studies emphasised that reporting success was also positively influenced by timely, useful feedback. This is probably a common human trait, and the lack of effective communication of results or recommendations can easily cool an individual's enthusiasm, as no one likes to work unnecessarily.

In conclusion, the success of reporting is proportional to low reporting burden and the accessibility to information. Thus, when designing an ideal system, cognitive- (understanding the importance) and emotional factors (enthusiasm, fear, satisfaction, etc.) as well as technological, organisational, and cultural aspects must be taken in consideration to facilitate easy and efficient reporting.

2. End note, wider context

By adopting the concept of learning from errors, medicine has taken the initial step to eliminate the "blame and shame" culture. However, there is still a long way ahead before openly admitting mistakes and capitalising on improvement potential of errors become the new norm. To build a new world, where the truth of "to err is human" is rediscovered, the full support of both mass and social media will also be needed. Presently, health-related news in the media can be frightening. Articles and interviews have never highlighted the fact that many important, forward moving changes in medicine were actually triggered by serious, even fatal errors. The attitude of the media and also the public opinion must be changed to acknowledge that it takes enormous courage and honour to openly admit mistakes instead of waiting out the consequences. Such moral strength may drive development in both individual and organisation level. Only such new, non-punitive but supportive systems are likely to be able to overcome deep-rooted emotional barriers such as fear, anxiety, guilt and appraise compassionate performance.

The authors of the chapter are also convinced that medical and media professionals alone will surely not be able to create this new system: the patients must to be given more weight in planning and design of care systems, as ultimately, we are working with them, not for them. In this new structure, patients (and caregivers) are more likely to receive high level of partnership-based carewith practitioners standing a better chance that a one-off error may not be ruining an otherwise immaculate long service careers of dedicated, talented professionals who dedicate their time and knowledge to helping others [16, 17].

3. Tasks and exercises

3.1 Exercise 1

What systems are in place in your setting to report harm? How are Datix, RIDDOR and Patient Liaison reports are collated and reported to you and your team? How many entries did you make in the adverse event log during the last year? How many should you have reported?

3.2 Exercise 2

Please ensure you are familiar with the risk assessment tools in your department? Are there any differences compared comparing to the above model? Is your tool better or worse than the tool above?

3.3 Exercise 3

How are adverse events dealt with in your organisation? How are the learning points communicated to your team?

3.4 Exercise 4

Are you aware of the effectiveness of root cause analysis within your organisation? If yes, what is the result?

4. Questions to consolidate knowledge

4.1 Question 1

How would you manage your team and in similar situation described in Box 2?

- Give the patient a call to explain and apologise
- Have a hot debrief to all involved staff
- Ask reflections from each members of staff
- Run a cause analysis and discuss results with all involved parties via a cold debrief
- Feed-back results to the whole team on an appropriate forum/channel

4.2 Question 2

What are the most common strategies to communicate errors and consequent recommendations to the team in your organisation?

- Mortality and Morbidity meetings
- A folder left in the staff room
- Circulars/newsletters

DOI: http://dx.doi.org/10.5772/intechopen.94126

Author details

Gabor Xantus[1]* and Laszlo Zavori[2]

1 Cardiff University, Cardiff, United Kingdom

2 Salisbury NHS Trust, Salisbury, United Kingdom

*Address all correspondence to: gabor.xantus@gmail.com

IntechOpen

© 2020 The Author(s). Licensee IntechOpen. This chapter is distributed under the terms of the Creative Commons Attribution License (http://creativecommons.org/licenses/by/3.0), which permits unrestricted use, distribution, and reproduction in any medium, provided the original work is properly cited.

References

[1] Vincent, Charles. Essence of patient Safety. Patient Safety. *BMJ Books*. Online: http://www.iarmm.org/IESRE2012May/Vincent_Essentials.pdf

[2] https://www.coverys.com/Knowledge-Center/a-dose-of-insight-emergency-department-risks

[3] https://resolution.nhs.uk/wp-content/uploads/2018/08/NHS-Resolution-Annual-Report-2017-2018.pdf

[4] Friesen, MA et al. Patient Safety and Quality: An Evidence-Based Handbook for Nurses. Chapter 34: Handoffs: Implications for Nurses 2008; 156–174

[5] Joint Commission: Patient Safety Systems Chapter 12, Sentinel Event Policy and RCA2. 2018; 41–49

[6] Root Cause Analysis. Institute for Health Care Improvement. Online. Available at: https://www.med.unc.edu/ihqi/resources/root-cause-analysis/

[7] Cause and effect diagram. Institute for Health Care Improvement. Online. Available at: http://www.ihi.org/resources/Pages/Tools/CauseandEffectDiagram.aspx

[8] 5 Whys: finding the root cause. Institute for Health Care Improvement. Online. Available at: http://www.ihi.org/resources/Pages/Tools/5-Whys-Finding-the-Root-Cause.aspx

[9] Murf HJ, Patel VL, Hripcsak G. et al. Detecting adverse events for patient safety research: a review of current methodologies. Journal of Biomedical Informatics 2003; 36(1): 131–143

[10] Hewitt T. és Chreim S. Fix and forget or fix and report: a qualitative study of tensions at the front line of incident reporting. BMJ Quality and Safety 2015; 24(5): 303–310.

[11] Cullen DL, Bates DW, Small SD. et al. The incident reporting system does not detect adverse drug events: a problem for quality improvement. Jt Comm J Qual Improv. 2011;(12):541–52

[12] Elder NC, Graham D, Brandt E. et al. Barriers and Motivators for Making Error Reports from Family Medicine Offices: A Report from the American Academy of Family Physicians National Research Network J Am Board fam Med. 2007;20(2):115–123

[13] Bayazidi S, Zarezadeh Y, Zamanzadeh V. et al. Medication Error Reporting Rate and its Barriers and Facilitators among Nurses Journal of Caring Science 2012; 1(4): 231–236

[14] Hartnell N, MacKinnon N, Sketris I. et al. Identifying, Understanding and Overcoming Barriers to Medication Error Reporting in Hospitals: A Focus Group Study. BMJ Qual Staf. 2012; 21 (5):361–368.

[15] Pooralaj J, Rezaie S, Aghighi N. Barriers to medical reporting. International Journal of Preventive Medicine 2015; (6):97–104

[16] Z. Wolf, R. Hughes. 2015 Patient Safety and Quality: An Evidence-Based Handbook for Nurses. Chapter 35. Error Reporting and Disclosure. 333–379

[17] Wu AW. Medical error: the second victim. BMJ 2018; (320):726–727

Section 3

Teamwork Implementation: Case Specifics

Chapter 8

Teamwork in a Surgical Department

Nikolai Ramadanov

Abstract

Teamwork is essential in surgery. A surgeon alone cannot fulfill his daily tasks. Surgical departments are divided into surgical teams: the surgical team in the operating theater, the surgical ward team, and the surgical emergency team. The common task of those teams is adequate patient care. The characteristics of team members describe necessary abilities such as: open communication, effective coordination skills, collaboration willingness, interdependency, mutual performance monitoring, backup behavior, adaptability, team orientation, and personality type. Team processes are recurring and ongoing short-term courses that occur in the team. The team developmental model separates the development of a team in four stages over a longer period of time. In the last stage, the team reaches the highest level of teamwork performance. Each team must be assessed for their nontechnical skills with team measurement tools. Surgical teams are insufficiently measured. There are possible disadvantages in teamwork, which must be considered and discussed versus the obvious benefits. Leadership is a process where the leading team member sets the direction for the others. There are different styles of leadership, whereby the dominant role of the leader is more or less pronounced. Leadership and teamwork are not contradicting characteristics of teams in the surgical department.

Keywords: teamwork, surgical department, leadership, surgical ward, operating theater

1. Introduction

Surgery is a major medical specialty that uses manual techniques to treat a pathological condition in patients. The classic surgical department of a hospital requires operating theaters with a professional surgical team to perform operations. A surgical team is made up of a surgeon, a surgeon's assistant, an anesthetist, a nurse anesthetist, a circulating nurse, and a surgical technologist. The surgical ward is occupied by those patients who have already undergone surgery, as well as those who are about to or might undergo surgery. These patients are cared for by the surgical ward team. A surgical ward team is composed of at least one surgeon and one surgical ward nurse. Furthermore, the classic surgical department often provides physicians for the treatment of emergency patients in the emergency room or supports emergency physicians with consultations in surgical emergency cases. Teams are obviously essential in all areas of the surgical department, since a single surgeon without additional personal support cannot work effectively.

2. Collaborative effort of a team to achieve a common goal

The collective effort of a group of people, a team, to achieve a common goal is called teamwork [1, 2]. Teamwork is used in any aspect of life where a group of people are working together for a common goal [1, 2]. Teamwork is commonly applied in sports, in industrial organizations, in school, in political parties and healthcare system. A team consists at least of two members. The team size is fixed, or it can vary depending upon the phase and complexity of the common goal. Still, every member must have a defined role within the team in order to be productive and to have a clear purpose within the team [3, 4]. The level of teamwork varies from low to high depending on the aspect of life it is applied. For example, soccer requires a high level of teamwork, whereas tennis requires significantly less teamwork. Good teamwork is linked to improved patient outcomes, better medical staff satisfaction and a reduced incidence of burnouts [5–7]. On the other hand, worse teamwork is linked to poorer patient outcomes due to adverse events, lack of coordination and higher costs [8–10]. Improvement of teamwork ability in operating theaters leads to reduced technical errors [11] and lower perioperative mortality [12]. However, most medical workers lack adequate training in teamwork in healthcare [13]. Some authors call for an emphasis on teamwork training in medical education [14]. In contrast to teamwork in acute cases, teamwork in nonacute patient cases is rarely trained. As chronic diseases place an increasing burden on health systems [15–17], the lack of team training needs to be adapted for long-term treatments [18].

Over the past decade, the efforts to perform better surgical performance increased [19]. Expectations for more transparency from operation results [20], better patient satisfaction and error reduction are rising [19]. In the context of our ongoing strive and expectations to improve health care, the facts paint a troubling picture. Operating theaters are a challenging area in the surgical department where human error can cause a great iatrogenic harm in a hospital [21, 22]. These unintentional adverse events have been reported to be up to 11% in British hospitals [23]. In 1999 the US Institute of Medicine estimated that 44,000 to 98,000 deaths occur in US hospitals annually, at least partially due to avoidable adverse events [24]. Up to two thirds of these events are due to surgical care [25, 26]. Communication errors have been identified as one of the main causes of these adverse events [24, 27]. Furthermore, e.g. it was reported that medication errors in emergency medicine of up to 31.1% were caused by surgeons and internists [28]. Communication problems in the emergency teams are discussed as a possible cause of incorrect drug administration. There have already been successes. E.g. promoting safety checklists has enhanced patient outcomes and reduced errors by improving teamwork [29]. In surgery in particular, the World Health Organization (WHO) has drawn up a safety checklist to enhance teamwork [30]. The improvement of teamwork, that is, nontechnical skills, might be one possible approach to achieving these goals.

The following pages are intended to give the reader an overview of teamwork in the surgical department. This chapter will clearly define the functions of the team members as well as different team constellations. It will describe the main characteristics of the team members. It will explain the team processes and the team development model. It will propose measurement tools for evaluating teamwork. It will discuss the benefits and drawbacks of teamwork and the necessity of strict leadership in the surgical department. It will propose approaches for a better patient outcome by improving teamwork.

3. Teams in the surgical department

Teamwork is essential in surgery. A surgeon alone cannot adequately fulfill his daily tasks, neither in the operating theater nor on the surgical ward. Classic surgical departments consist of several different types of surgical teams with different tasks in everyday hospital life. The common task of those teams is the adequate care for their patients. In general, we can distinguish between three important teams. There is the surgical team in the operating theater, the surgical ward team and the emergency surgical team.

3.1 The surgical team in operating theater

The operating team in the operating room consists of a surgeon, an anesthetist, a surgeon's assistant, a nurse anesthetist, a circulating nurse, and a surgical technologist. There is a clearly structured hierarchy in the team in the order of the members just mentioned. The tasks of each member are clearly defined. The level of leadership is particularly pronounced in the surgical team in operating theater [31]. The work of the surgical team has a direct impact on patient outcome. The privilege and burden of decision-making is primarily focused on the surgeon. The overall environment in the operating theater, the performance and the collaboration between the individual team members largely depend on the behavior, knowledge and interpersonal skills of the surgeon. The level of stress in the operating room is much higher compared to teams in other areas of life. It is therefore of the utmost importance that every member, apart from the self-evident technical competence and preparation, has a high level of teamwork and reliability. The surgical team in the operating theater is a very well-coordinated and professional team. Beginners are subjected to a comprehensive and strictly controlled training until they reach the stage of being able to master their part of the task with confidence. Frequent changes to the members of the core team must be avoided. They negatively affect surgical performance [32]. Frequent changes of core team members must be avoided. They have a negative influence on surgical performance [32].

3.1.1 Surgeon

The surgeon is a physician with completed residency in surgery, who possesses all certifications required for practicing general or specialized surgery. He often is specialized in a particular area of surgery such as abdominal surgery, trauma surgery, pediatric surgery, vascular surgery, thoracic surgery, plastic surgery and cardiac surgery. The task of the surgeon is primarily to lead the operation and the surgical team. Furthermore, the surgeon needs to have full knowledge of the operational procedure and the instruments required. Especially the surgeon bears the responsibility for the successful outcome of the operation. Therefore, his leadership role in such an important team brings him advantages and a great burden at the same time.

3.1.2 Anesthetist

The anesthetist is a physician with completed residency in anesthesiology, who possesses all certifications required for performing narcosis and local anesthesia. The professional interest and responsibility of the anesthetist extends to the patient's overall health before, during and after surgery. In addition to ensuring a painless operation, the most important task of the anesthetist is to monitor and maintain the vital functions of the patient during the operation. Constant collegial communication and feedback in both directions is absolutely necessary between anesthetist and surgeon. Criticism of communication difficulties comes from both sides.

3.1.3 Surgical assistant

The role of the surgical assistant is held by different members of the team. On the one hand, resident physicians assist in operations as part of their surgical training, on the other hand, this role can be assumed by registered nurse first assistants. The surgical assistant receives clear and unambiguous instructions from the surgeon. The participation of the surgical assistant must not be limited to a mere passive presence at the operating table. It is an active responsible assignment with constant communication with the surgeon leading the operation.

3.1.4 Nurse anesthetist

The nurse anesthetist is an advanced practice registered nurse. She supports the anesthetist before, during and after surgery. The nurse anesthetist receives clear and unambiguous instructions from the anesthetist. Constant communication and feedback with the anesthetist is absolutely necessary.

3.1.5 Surgical technologist

Surgical technologists are trained in numerous types of operations. They are able to assume the next steps in the operational procedure in order to provide the surgeon with the necessary instruments without delay. This helps the surgeon to focus adequately on surgery. The surgical technologists are registered nurses or other medical staff with an appropriate education. They receive clear and unambiguous instructions from the surgeon. Constant communication and feedback with the surgeon is absolutely necessary.

3.1.6 Circulating nurse

Circulating nurses take care of the procurement of instruments and surgical accessories. The circulating nurse receives from the surgical technologist or from the surgeon directly. Constant communication and feedback with the surgical technologist is absolutely necessary.

3.2 The surgical ward team

The surgical ward team consists of at least one surgeon and one nurse. The team is led by a surgical consultant or a surgical registrar [33]. The surgical registrar must have the guaranteed possibility to consult the chief surgeon for pending questions. This team conducts the daily ward round of the patients in the surgical ward and takes care of the resulting ward work. The surgical ward round is a complex process [33]. Sometimes it lasts several hours until all parameters in every patient case are assessed completely [33]. It is advantageous if the individual members of the surgical ward team do not change too often, e.g. for at least a week, as this will interrupt the continuity of the individual patient cases. Wound care, dressing changes and wraps must always be made by both the surgeon and the nurse. Otherwise mandatory hygienic rules and sterility cannot be adhered to. Once again, constant collegial communication and feedback in both directions between surgeon and nurse is absolutely necessary for the team.

3.3 The emergency surgical team

During normal course of action in the emergency room, the emergency surgical team consists of a physician, who is a surgeon or an emergency physician with a background surgical consultant, and a registered emergency nurse. When treating polytraumatized patients, the general or trauma surgeon is the trauma leader. The shock room supply follows ATLS guidelines [34]. Since the polytraumatized patient is in life-threatening condition, the surgeon's leadership role becomes even more important than in surgical team constellations in other areas. Having the decision-making power, the surgeon bears the greatest responsibility for the patient's outcome. The surgeon depends on a competent and reliable team to achieve the common goal. However, teamwork is a key component to the success of the emergency surgery team.

4. Characteristics of team members

The characteristics of the team members describe necessary abilities, which are a prerequisite for the proper functioning of the team. A sufficient level of professional and technical competence and preparation is a matter of course. However, nontechnical skills are just as important for teamwork.

Open communication and effective coordination skills are required to avoid conflicts, confusion and overstepping boundaries or to resolve existing conflicts healthy [35]. Collaboration willingness is required to complete tasks on time and to share the workload fairly. Furthermore, a high level of interdependency is required to maintain trust, reliability and risk taking. Mutual performance monitoring describes the ability to understand the intentions, roles, and responsibilities of other team members [36]. In this way members can closely monitor performance of others for the purpose of common goal [37]. Backup behavior describes the ability to look after the needs of other team members and to ensure balance during times of increased workload [36]. Adaptability describes the ability of team members to adapt their work to feedback from other team members in order to achieve the common goal [38]. This characteristic requires flexibility. Every team member must be able to adequately response to changing conditions [36]. Team orientation describes the ability to prioritize team goals over individual goals and to respect different opinions [37, 39, 40].

The motivation of the team members has to be present and preserved. Clear and attainable goals must be set. Satisfactory education and career opportunities must be promoted for residents and other team members. Further requirements are the willingness to balanced member contributions, mutual support, effort, and cohesion [41]. The personality type of the team members is a characteristic that cannot be trained. It can only be adjusted to a certain extent. During the hiring of the team member, care must be taken to ensure that they complement and enrich the team and that their specific personality type suits the team. Unsuitable personality type constellation in the team has to be corrected by cancelation or rotations of team members. Here, a proven method of measuring teamwork in people wanting to join a team can help out. The knowledge, skills, and abilities teamwork test (KSA) was introduced in 1994 by Stevens [42]. In a 35-point test it assesses 14 individual KSA requirements for teamwork. The KSA focuses on team-oriented situations, which makes it suitable for evaluating teamwork and team-specific behavior, determining the level of teamwork and finding ways to improve communication.

5. Team processes in the surgical department

Team processes are recurring and ongoing short-term courses that occur in the team. The following specific teamwork processes are grouped into three categories: transition processes, action processes and interpersonal processes [43, 44]. Consciously going through these processes by the team leads to a general improvement in performance by improving collaboration, coordination, and communication of the team members [45]. Action processes occur when the team takes tangible steps to achieve their goals. The progress toward the goals is monitored by responsible team members. Transition processes take place between periods of action. During the transition process, the team assesses its overall performance. The team members give feedback to each other and try to improve the upcoming action process. The interpersonal process is an ongoing process in which team members have to communicate all their positive and/or negative opinions about other team members or about the team's performance.

6. Team developmental model

The team developmental model proposes to separate the development of a team in four stages over a longer period of time: forming, storming, norming, and performing [46]. There are different levels of teamwork in each stage. The forming stage is characterized by mistrust, lack of risk-taking, approach and avoidance attempts of the new team members. There is an internal conflict between members who seek their place among themselves. This stage has a low level of teamwork performance. The storming stage is the stage of deeper conflicts. There is competition for power and authority between team members. This stage has a varying level of teamwork performance, which is predictive for the future of the team. The norming stage is characterized by rising levels of interdependence, team spirit and reliability. This stage has a high level of teamwork performance. The performing stage is the last stage of team development. It is characterized by a satisfactory environment in which the team is able to accomplish its tasks most effectively and successfully. This stage has the highest level of teamwork performance.

7. Measuring and training of teamwork

Each team must be regularly assessed for their nontechnical skills. The causes of good and bad team results must be identified in the characteristics of the team members. Feedback must be given to all team members. The identified weaknesses or strengths in the characteristics of the team members can thus be corrected or promoted. To implement this task, tools had to be developed that allow nontechnical skills of a team to be measured. Numerous such measurement tools have so far been developed for teams in general and have been improved over time. With the increasing awareness that teamwork is fundamental to the outcome of surgical patients [47], progress has also been made in measurement of nontechnical surgical team skills over the past decade. However, experience shows that in practice surgical teams are insufficiently and inconsistently measured [47]. The possibility of training teamwork with serious improvement of the team performance is questionable. While some authors recommend regular team training [14, 48], a systematic review of literature from 2011 with 1036 identified relevant abstracts and 14 articles (four randomized studies and 10 nonrandomized studies) analyzed in detail came to the conclusion that evidence for the technical or clinical benefits of teamwork training in medicine is insufficient [49]. Another systematic review of literature from 2018 stated that there is insufficient evidence to support the hypothesis that teamwork training interventions improve patient outcomes [19]. One could conclude from this that the personality type of the team members plays a very important role, as this is the main characteristic that can hardly be changed or trained. Candidates wishing to join the team must therefore be carefully screened for their suitability with the rest of the team.

7.1 Measuring tools for the surgical team

Current literature shows that teamwork disruptions, communication errors, cultural and hierarchical barriers lead to safety deficiencies in the operating rooms [50–53]. Furthermore, a systematic review of the literature from 2012 with 28 included studies showed a strong correlation between teamwork failure and technical errors during surgery [54]. A control instrument was required. Several tools have been developed to evaluate teamwork in operating theaters based on direct observation or video analysis [50, 55–63]. In a current systematic review of 2121 searched references and 14 studies included, two assessment tools were identified to measure effectively the nontechnical skills of the surgical team in the operating theater: The Observational Teamwork Assessment for Surgery (OTAS) and Operating Theater Team Non-Technical Skills Assessment Tool (NOTECHS) [47]. The criticism of both tools is that they rely on the questionable assumption that the team performance equals the sum of performances of the team members [47]. The Observational Teamwork Assessment for Surgery was introduced in 2009 by Sevdalis [55] and validated in 2010 by Hull [56]. OTAS consists of 15 items with a 7-point scale and assesses teamwork-related task checklists and teamwork-related behaviors [55]. The validity and reliability of the NOTECHS tool was demonstrated in live operating theater environments in 2009 by Mishra [57]. The tool was restructured and improved in 2014 by Robertson [57]. The new NOTECHS II tool offers a higher level of precision and a higher measuring sensitivity [58]. Another systematic review of iterature from 2015 with 25 studies included concluded that the Nontechnical Skills for Surgeons (NOTSS) assessment was the tool with the highest level of validity, reliability, and acceptability [64]. The NOTSS assesses situation awareness, decision-making, communication, teamwork, and leadership in a 4-point numeric scale system [65, 66]. A systematic review of literature from 2013 indicated that safety checklists are beneficial for teamwork and communication in the operating theater [67]. This may be one mechanism through which patient outcomes are improved [67]. The results of another systematic review and meta-analysis from 2014 with 19 included studies found that surgical safety checklists improve teamwork and communication, reduce morbidity and mortality [68].

7.2 Measuring tools for the surgical ward team

Teamwork in the surgical ward is as important as in the operating theater. In an assessment of patient risks associated with poor communication in surgical care the following problems were detected: communication during the surgical ward round is often limited between patient and physician, with nurses making little contribution [69]. Nurses sometimes have important additional information about patients. Unlike physicians, they monitor patients' daily activities. Therefore, only surgical ward rounds with an integrated assessment by different professional groups, including nurses, allow a complete collection of the important and necessary patient information [69]. Up to two thirds of the deadly events in hospitals are due to surgical care [25, 26]. Communication errors have been identified as the main cause of these adverse events [24, 27]. A study on surgical treatment errors due to communication breakdown showed that their occurrence is equally distributed across the continuum of care, before, during and after surgery [51]. Despite this knowledge about the distribution of adverse events, there is sparse literature on the measurement of teamwork quality in the surgical ward. Filling this large gap in science will show at which points in the surgical ward improvements in teamwork are necessary. In 2019, Krishnamohan introduced a surgical ward round checklist to monitor documentation [33]. It is claimed to improve communication between team members in the surgical ward team [33]. In 2014, Hull introduced a combined assessment toolkit for technical and nontechnical team skills in surgical ward care [70]. It consists of a novel clinical checklist for ward care (Clinical Skills Assessment for Ward Care); a novel team assessment scale for ward rounds (Teamwork Skills Assessment for Ward Care); and a revised version of a physician-patient interaction scale (Physician-Patient Interaction Global Rating Scale) [70]. It provides a systematic assessment of the quality and safety of surgical care and can be used to check and train residents' skills and performance.

7.3 Measuring tools for the emergency surgical team

The surgical team in the emergency room is often exposed to critical situations. Managing patients in a life-threatening condition is probably the greatest responsibility of medical staff. These teams often consist of interdisciplinary medical staff which is exposed to the challenge to work simultaneously on the treatment of critically ill patients [71]. Wrong decisions quickly lead to fatal consequences. For this reason, in addition to necessary knowledge and experience, strict leadership of the team is required. Only then can clear and quick decisions be made and unambiguous instructions given to the team. Leadership skills are highlighted in advanced life support training and have shown beneficial results in simulated and clinical resuscitation scenarios [72]. A study of 106 adult resuscitation team events with three or more team members over a 10-month period found a need for leadership training [73]. Emergency teams must develop their leadership skills through training and reflective debriefing [73]. Nevertheless, teamwork is indispensable again. A promising way to improve quality in emergency teams is to use nontechnical skills that aim to address human factors by improving leadership, communication, and decision-making [72]. Assessments to evaluate the nontechnical skills of the team are essential to reduce medical errors and improve team performance [71]. In a systematic review of literature from 2016 10 assessment tools for nontechnical skills of hospital action teams were identified [71]. Unfortunately, the validity of these assessment tools to measure the nontechnical performance is limited [71]. A feasible, valid, and reliable measuring tool is the Team Emergency Assessment Measure (TEAM) [73].

8. Benefits and disadvantages of teamwork

Despite the numerous studies that have found advantages in the use of nontechnical skills in surgery, possible disadvantages are still being discussed [74, 75]. Over-focusing on teamwork can prevent teams from peaking. On the one hand, this can affect the whole team or, more often, individual team members who, like the faster animals in a moving herd, wait for the slower ones. In this way more competitive and talented team members can be disadvantaged in favor of the team and their development can be slowed down. One can certainly imagine that the desire and pursuit of professional self-actualization and even showing off is more strongly expressed among surgeons than among other groups of physicians. Forced commitment to teamwork might reduce the autonomy and individualism of some team members. In other cases, the workload is unevenly distributed, with some team members doing more work and others less. Therefore, the aim of the team leader and of all team members must be to avoid such unfair events. All of these events are possible reasons for conflict in the team. The resulting conflicts prevent the team from achieving the common goal. These potential problems in the team should be considered. A team needs to create conditions for healthy team competition. This can help keep team members motivated, outperform the team average and not suppress individual talents. Again, taking into account the professional development of individual team members must not impair the team cooperation, as it is known that team cooperation is more often associated with very successful and effective teams [76, 77].

Still, the distinct advantages in teamwork in the surgical department must be emphasized. A combined problem-solving effort of the team has surely more potential than an individual [78]. Another advantage of teamwork is building relationships. The pursuit of a common goal leads to greater cohesion, which improves the team's performance [43, 78]. Distinct individual qualities of a team member can also be advantageous in case that the knowledge and skills are offered to improve other team members.

9. Leadership and teamwork

Team leadership describes the ability to coordinate team activities, to distribute tasks fairly, to evaluate performance, to provide feedback and in this way to enhance the team performance [37, 39]. Leadership is a process where the leading team member sets the direction for one or more team members and helps them improve their performance [79]. Positive leadership skills lead to better satisfaction of the medical staff, higher motivation of team members, increased staff retention, and improved performance [80–83]. Beneficial team leadership leads to increased patient satisfaction and reduced adverse events [84–86].

There are different styles of leadership [87], whereby the dominant role of the leader is more or less pronounced. The style of leadership indicates the level of authority of the team leader. Under strict leadership there is less freedom and leeway for subordinate team members. Strict leadership is based on a pronounced hierarchy in the team, led by an authoritarian leader with subordinate followers. On the other hand, servant leadership is a style in leadership where leaders serve their followers [88–90]. Servant leaders try to build a stable organization, bring out the best performance and serve the team [91]. A detailed comparison of lean and servant leadership is given in a systematic review of literature of 29 articles [92]. A systematic review of literature with 18 articles included found that leadership styles were strongly correlated with quality in care, both for the patients and medical staff [93]. Finally, leadership and teamwork must not be seen as contradicting characteristics of teams in the surgical department. Strict leadership does not automatically exclude the need for a functioning team. Every style of leadership and even strict leadership depends on the team members and on their differently led team.

10. Conclusion

Teamwork is essential in surgery. A surgeon alone cannot adequately fulfill his daily tasks, neither in the operating theater nor in the surgical ward nor in the emergency department (**Table 1**). The teamwork, that is, nontechnical skills,

Key points	Remarks/explanations
Types of surgical teams	
Surgical team in operating theater	Consists of a surgeon, an anesthetist, a surgeon's assistant, a nurse anesthetist, a circulating nurse, and a surgical technologist
Surgical ward team	Consists of at least one surgeon and one nurse
Emergency surgical team	The general or trauma surgeon is the trauma leader, when treating polytraumatized patients
Characteristics of team members	
Communication and coordination	Required to avoid conflicts, confusion, and overstepping boundaries
Collaboration	Required to complete tasks on time and to share the workload fairly
Interdependency	Required to maintain trust, reliability, and risk taking
Mutual performance monitoring	Ability to understand the intentions, roles, and responsibilities of other team members
Backup behavior	Ability to look after the needs of other team members
Adaptability	Ability to adapt the work to feedback from other team members
Team orientation	Ability to prioritize team goals and to respect different opinions
Personality type	Cannot be trained; it can only be adjusted to a certain extent
Team processes	
Action process	When the team takes tangible steps to achieve their goals
Transition process	Between two action processes
Interpersonal process	Ongoing communication about positive and/or negative opinions or about the team's performance
Team developmental model	
Forming	Internal conflict between team members; low level of teamwork performance
Storming	Deeper conflicts due to competition for power and authority between team members; varying level of teamwork performance
Norming	Rising levels of interdependence, team spirit and reliability; high level of teamwork performance
Performing	Team is able to accomplish its tasks most successfully; highest level of teamwork performance
Measuring tools	
OTAS	Teamwork assessment tool in operating theater
NOTECHS	Teamwork assessment tool in operating theater
NOTSS	Teamwork assessment tool in operating theater
Tool for technical and nontechnical skills in surgical ward care	Combined assessment toolkit for technical and nontechnical team skills in surgical ward care
TEAM	Measuring tool for teamwork in emergency
KSA	Knowledge, skills, and abilities test measuring teamwork in people wanting to join a team

Table 1.
Summary table of important information.

DOI: http://dx.doi.org/10.5772/intechopen.93698

of teams in the surgical department has an obvious impact on patient outcome. The privilege and burden of decision-making is primarily focused on the surgeon. The performance of the team members depends on the behavior, knowledge, and interpersonal and leadership skills of the surgeon as a team leader. Every team leader depends on his team members. Leadership and teamwork must not be seen as contradicting characteristics of the teams in the surgical department. Both are necessary for the surgical department to function. Each team must be regularly assessed for their nontechnical skills. The causes of good and bad team results must be identified in the characteristics of the team members. Feedback must be given to all team members. The identified weaknesses or strengths in the characteristics of the team members can thus be corrected or promoted. To implement this task, tools had to be developed that allow nontechnical skills of a team to be measured. Two assessment tools are recommended to measure the nontechnical skills of the surgical team in the operating theater: The Observational Teamwork Assessment for Surgery (OTAS) and Operating Theater Team Non-Technical Skills Assessment Tool (NOTECHS). There is a reliable combined assessment tool to measure technical and nontechnical team skills in the surgical ward team. It consists of a novel clinical checklist for ward care (Clinical Skills Assessment for Ward Care); a novel team assessment scale for wards rounds (Teamwork Skills Assessment for Ward Care); and a revised version of a physician-patient interaction scale (Physician-Patient Interaction Global Rating Scale). The Team Emergency Assessment Measure (TEAM) can be used as a measuring tool for emergency surgical teams. Current literature shows that teamwork training interventions do not improve patient outcomes significantly. The personality type of the team members seems to play a very important role, as this is the main characteristic that can hardly be changed or trained. Candidates wishing to join the team must therefore be carefully screened for their suitability with the rest of the team. This is where the Teamwork Test (KSA) of knowledge, skills, and abilities can be helpful as a proven method of measuring teamwork in people who want to join a team. Frequent changes to the members of the core surgical team should be avoided, since the surgical team is a very well-coordinated and professional team. Despite the numerous studies that have found advantages in the use of nontechnical skills in surgery, possible disadvantages are still being discussed. Over-focusing on teamwork can prevent team members from peaking. More competitive and talented team members might be disadvantaged in favor of the team and their development can be slowed down. Forced commitment to teamwork might reduce the autonomy and individualism of some team members. A team needs to create conditions for healthy team competition. This can help keep team members motivated, outperform the team average and not suppress individual talents. Still, the distinct advantages in teamwork in the surgical department must be emphasized. A combined problem-solving effort of the team has surely more potential than an individual. The pursuit of a common goal leads to greater cohesion, which improves the team's performance. Distinct individual qualities of a team member can also be advantageous in case that the knowledge and skills are offered to improve other team members. Once again, teamwork is essential in surgery.

Author details

Nikolai Ramadanov
Center for Emergency Medicine, University Hospital of Jena, Jena, Germany

*Address all correspondence to: nikolai.ramadanov@gmail.com

IntechOpen

© 2020 The Author(s). Licensee IntechOpen. This chapter is distributed under the terms of the Creative Commons Attribution License (http://creativecommons.org/licenses/by/3.0), which permits unrestricted use, distribution, and reproduction in any medium, provided the original work is properly cited.

References

[1] Salas E, Cooke NJ, Rosen MA. On teams, teamwork, and team performance: Discoveries and developments. Human Factors. 2008;**50**(3):540-547. DOI: 10.1518/001872008X288457

[2] Driskell JE, Salas E, Driskell T. Foundations of teamwork and collaboration. The American Psychologist. 2018;**73**(4):334-348. DOI: 10.1037/amp0000241

[3] Chang A, Bordia P, Duck J. Punctuated equilibrium and linear progression: Toward a new understanding of group development. Academy of Management Journal. 2003;**46**(1):106-117. DOI: 10.2307/30040680

[4] Gersick C. Revolutionary change theories: A multilevel exploration of the punctuated equilibrium paradigm. Academy of Management Review. 1991;**16**:10-16. DOI: 10.5465/amr.1991.4278988

[5] Helfrich CD, Dolan ED, Simonetti J, Reid RJ, Joos S, Wakefield BJ, et al. Elements of team-based care in a patient-centered medical home are associated with lower burnout among VA primary care employees. Journal of General Internal Medicine. 2014;**29**(2):659-666. DOI: 10.1007/s11606-013-2702-z

[6] Gittell JH, Fairfield KM, Bierbaum B, Head W, Jackson R, Kelly M, et al. Impact of relational coordination on quality of care, postoperative pain and functioning, and length of stay: A nine-hospital study of surgical patients. Medical Care. 2000;**38**(8):807-819. DOI: 10.1097/00005650-200008000-00005

[7] Lemieux-Charles L, McGuire WL. What do we know about health care team effectiveness? A review of the literature. Medical Care Research and Review. 2006;**63**(3):263-300. DOI: 10.1177/1077558706287003

[8] Petersen LA, Brennan TA, O'Neil AC, Cook EF, Lee TH. Does house staff discontinuity of care increase the risk for preventable adverse events? Annals of Internal Medicine. 1994;**121**(11): 866-872. DOI: 10.7326/0003-4819-121-11-199412010-00008

[9] Williams RG, Silverman R, Schwind C, Fortune JB, Sutyak J, Horvath KD, et al. Surgeon information transfer and communication: Factors affecting quality and efficiency of inpatient care. Annals of Surgery. 2007;**245**(2):159-169. DOI: 10.1097/01.sla.0000242709.28760.56

[10] Mazzocco K, Petitti DB, Fong KT, Bonacum D, Brookey J, Graham S, et al. Surgical team behaviors and patient outcomes. American Journal of Surgery. 2009;**197**(5):678-685. DOI: 10.1016/j.amjsurg.2008.03.002

[11] McCulloch P, Mishra A, Handa A, Dale T, Hirst G, Catchpole K. The effects of aviation-style non-technical skills training on technical performance and outcome in the operating theatre. Quality & Safety in Health Care. 2009;**18**(2):109-115. DOI: 10.1136/qshc.2008.032045

[12] Neily J, Mills PD, Young-Xu Y, et al. Association between implementation of a medical team training program and surgical mortality. Journal of the American Medical Association. 2010;**304**(15):1693-1700. DOI: 10.1001/jama.2010.1506

[13] Dzau VJ, McClellan M, McGinnis JM. Vital directions for health and health care: An initiative of the National Academy of Medicine [published correction appears in JAMA. 2018 Dec 25;320(24):2602]. Journal

of the American Medical Association. 2016;**316**(7):711-712. DOI: 10.1001/jama.2016.10692

[14] Association of Program Directors in Internal Medicine, Fitzgibbons JP, Bordley DR, Berkowitz LR, Miller BW, Henderson MC. Redesigning residency education in internal medicine: A position paper from the Association of Program Directors in Internal Medicine. Annals of Internal Medicine. 2006;**144**(12):920-926. DOI: 10.7326/0003-4819-144-12-200606200-00010

[15] Anderson G, Horvath J. The growing burden of chronic disease in America. Public Health Reports. 2004;**119**(3):263-270. DOI: 10.1016/j.phr.2004.04.005

[16] Thorpe KE, Howard DH. The rise in spending among medicare beneficiaries: The role of chronic disease prevalence and changes in treatment intensity. Health Affairs (Millwood). 2006;**25**(5):w378-w388. DOI: 10.1377/hlthaff.25.w378

[17] Emanuel EJ. Where are the health care cost savings? Journal of the American Medical Association. 2012;**307**(1):39-40. DOI: 10.1001/jama.2011.1927

[18] Marlow SL, Hughes AM, Sonesh SC, et al. A systematic review of team training in health care: Ten questions. Joint Commission Journal on Quality and Patient Safety. 2017;**43**(4):197-204. DOI: 10.1016/j.jcjq.2016.12.004

[19] Sun R, Marshall DC, Sykes MC, Maruthappu M, Shalhoub J. The impact of improving teamwork on patient outcomes in surgery: A systematic review. International Journal of Surgery. 2018;**53**:171-177. DOI: 10.1016/j.ijsu.2018.03.044

[20] Calland JF, Guerlain S, Adams RB, Tribble CG, Foley E, Chekan EG. A systems approach to surgical safety. Surgical Endoscopy. 2002;**16**(6):1005-1015. DOI: 10.1007/s00464-002-8509-3

[21] Leape LL. Error in medicine. JAMA. 1994;**272**:1851-1857

[22] Lear R, Riga C, Godfrey AD, Falaschetti E, Cheshire NJ, Van Herzeele I, et al. Multicentre observational study of surgical system failures in aortic procedures and their effect on patient outcomes. The British Journal of Surgery. 2016;**103**(11):1467-1475. DOI: 10.1002/bjs.10275

[23] Vincent C, Neale G, Woloshynowych M. Adverse events in British hospitals: Preliminary retrospective record review [published correction appears in BMJ. 2001 Jun 9;322(7299):1395]. BMJ. 2001;**322**(7285):517-519. DOI: 10.1136/bmj.322.7285.517

[24] Kohn L. To err is human: An interview with the Institute of Medicine's Linda Kohn. Joint Commission Journal on Quality Improvement. 2000;**26**(4):227-234

[25] Thomas EJ, Studdert DM, Burstin HR, Orav EJ, Zeena T, Williams EJ, et al. Incidence and types of adverse events and negligent care in Utah and Colorado. Medical Care. 2000;**38**(3):261-271. DOI: 10.1097/00005650-200003000-00003

[26] Gawande AA, Thomas EJ, Zinner MJ, Brennan TA. The incidence and nature of surgical adverse events in Colorado and Utah in 1992. Surgery. 1999;**126**(1):66-75. DOI: 10.1067/msy.1999.98664

[27] Leape LL, Brennan TA, Laird N, Lawthers AG, Localio AR, Barnes BA, et al. The nature of adverse events in hospitalized patients. Results of the Harvard Medical Practice Study II. The New England Journal of Medicine. 1991;**324**(6):377-384. DOI: 10.1056/NEJM199102073240605

[28] Ramadanov N, Klein R, Schumann U, Aguilar ADV, Behringer W. Factors, influencing medication errors in prehospital care: A retrospective observational study. Medicine (Baltimore). 2019;**98**(49):e18200. DOI: 10.1097/MD.0000000000018200

[29] Ko HC, Turner TJ, Finnigan MA. Systematic review of safety checklists for use by medical care teams in acute hospital settings--Limited evidence of effectiveness. BMC Health Services Research. 2011;**11**:211. DOI: 10.1186/1472-6963-11-211

[30] Haynes AB, Weiser TG, Berry WR, Lipsitz SR, Breizat AHS, Dellinger EP, et al. A surcal safety checklist to reduce morbidity and mortality in a global population. The New England Journal of Medicine. 2009;**360**(5):491-499. DOI: 10.1056/NEJMsa0810119

[31] Stone JL, Aveling EL, Frean M, Shields MC, Wright C, Gino F, et al. Effective leadership of surgical teams: A mixed methods study of surgeon behaviors and functions. The Annals of Thoracic Surgery. 2017;**104**(2):530-537. DOI: 10.1016/j.athoracsur.2017.01.021

[32] Zheng B, Panton ON, Al-Tayeb TA. Operative length independently affected by surgical team size: Data from 2 Canadian hospitals. Canadian Journal of Surgery. 2012;**55**(6):371-376. DOI: 10.1503/cjs.011311

[33] Krishnamohan N, Maitra I, Shetty VD. The surgical ward round checklist: Improving patient safety and clinical documentation. Journal of Multidisciplinary Healthcare. 2019;**12**:789-794. DOI: 10.2147/JMDH.S178896

[34] ATLS Subcommittee, American College of Surgeons' Committee on Trauma, International ATLS Working Group. Advanced trauma life support (ATLS®): The ninth edition. Journal of Trauma and Acute Care Surgery. 2013;**74**(5):1363-1366. DOI: 10.1097/TA.0b013e31828b82f5

[35] Tørring B, Gittell JH, Laursen M, Rasmussen BS, Sørensen EE. Communication and relationship dynamics in surgical teams in the operating room: An ethnographic study. BMC Health Services Research. 2019;**19**(1):528. DOI: 10.1186/s12913-019-4362-0

[36] Leasure EL, Jones RR, Meade LB, et al. There is no "i" in teamwork in the patient-centered medical home: Defining teamwork competencies for academic practice. Academic Medicine. 2013;**88**(5):585-592. DOI: 10.1097/ACM.0b013e31828b0289

[37] Baker DP, Day R, Salas E. Teamwork as an essential component of high-reliability organizations. Health Services Research. 2006;**41**(4 pt 2):1576-1598. DOI: 10.1111/j.1475-6773.2006.00566.x

[38] Stout RJ, Salas E, Fowlkes JE. Enhancing teamwork in complex environments through team training. Group Dynamics: Theory, Research, and Practice. 1997;**1**:169-182. DOI: 10.1037/1089-2699.1.2.169

[39] Baker DP, Salas E, King H, Battles J, Barach P. The role of teamwork in the professional education of physicians: Current status and assessment recommendations. Joint Commission Journal on Quality and Patient Safety. 2005;**31**:185-202. DOI: 10.1016/s1553-7250(05)31025-7

[40] Driskell JE, Salas E. Collective behavior and team performance. Human Factors. 1992;**34**:277-288. DOI: 10.1177/001872089203400303

[41] Hoegl M, Gemuenden HG. Teamwork quality and the success of innovative projects: A theoretical concept and empirical evidence. Organization Science.

2001;**12**(4):435-449. DOI: 10.1287/orsc.12.4.435.10635

[42] Stevens M, Campion M. The knowledge, skill, and ability requirements for teamwork: Implications of human resource management. Journal of Management. 1994;**20**(2):503-530. DOI: 10.1177/014920639402000210

[43] Marks MA, Mathieu JE, Zacaro SJA. Temporally based framework and taxonomy of team processes. Academy of Management Review. 2001;**26**(3): 356-376. DOI: 10.2307/259182

[44] LePine JA, Piccolo RF, Jackson CL, Mathieu JE, Saul JRA. Meta-analysis of teamwork processes: Tests of a multidimensional model and relationships with team effectiveness criteria. Personnel Psychology. 2008;**61**(2):273-307. DOI: 10.1111/j.1744-6570.2008.00114.x

[45] Cattani G, Ferriani S, Mariani M, Mengoli S. Tackling the 'Galácticos' effect: Team familiarity and the performance of star-studded projects. Industrial and Corporate Change. 2013;**22**(6):1629-1662. DOI: 10.1093/icc/dtt001

[46] Tuckman B. Developmental sequence in small groups. Psychological Bulletin. 1965;**63**(6):384-399. DOI: 10.1037/h0022100

[47] Etherington N, Larrigan S, Liu H, Wu M, Sullivan KJ, Jung J, et al. Measuring the teamwork performance of operating room teams: A systematic review of assessment tools and their measurement properties. Journal of Interprofessional Care. 2019;**22**:1-9. DOI: 10.1080/13561820.2019.1702931

[48] Forse R, Bramble D, McQuillan R. Team training can improve operating room performance. Surgery. 2011;**150**(4):771-778. DOI: 10.1016/j.surg.2011.07.076

[49] McCulloch P, Rathbone J, Catchpole K. Interventions to improve teamwork and communications among healthcare staff. The British Journal of Surgery. 2011;**98**(4):469-479. DOI: 10.1002/bjs.7434

[50] Lingard L, Reznick R, Espin S, Regehr G, DeVito I. Team communications in the operating room: Talk patterns, sites of tension, and implications for novices. Academic Medicine. 2002;**77**(3):232-237. DOI: 10.1097/00001888-200203000-00013

[51] Greenberg CC, Regenbogen SE, Studdert DM, Lipsitz SR, Rogers SO, Zinner MJ, et al. Patterns of communication breakdowns resulting in injury to surgical patients. Journal of the American College of Surgeons. 2007;**204**(4):533-540. DOI: 10.1016/j.jamcollsurg.2007.01.010

[52] Rosenstein AH, O'Daniel M. Impact and implications of disruptive behavior in the perioperative arena. Journal of the American College of Surgeons. 2006;**203**(1):96-105. DOI: 10.1016/j.jamcollsurg.2006.03.027

[53] Kennedy TJ, Regehr G, Baker GR, Lingard L. Preserving professional credibility: Grounded theory study of medical trainees' requests for clinical support. BMJ. 2009;**338**:b128. DOI: 10.1136/bmj.b128

[54] Hull L, Arora S, Aggarwal R, Darzi A, Vincent C, Sevdalis N. The impact of nontechnical skills on technical performance in surgery: A systematic review. Journal of the American College of Surgeons. 2012;**214**(2):214-230. DOI: 10.1016/j.jamcollsurg.2011.10.016

[55] Sevdalis N, Lyons M, Healey AN, Undre S, Darzi A, Vincent CA. Observational teamwork assessment for surgery: Construct validation with expert versus novice raters. Annals of Surgery. 2009;**249**(6):1047-1051. DOI: 10.1097/SLA.0b013e3181a50220

[56] Hull L, Arora S, Kassab E, Kneebone R, Sevdalis N. Observational teamwork assessment for surgery: Content validation and tool refinement. Journal of the American College of Surgeons. 2011;**212**(2):234. e2435-243.e2435. DOI: 10.1016/j.jamcollsurg.2010.11.001

[57] Mishra A, Catchpole K, McCulloch P. The Oxford NOTECHS system: Reliability and validity of a tool for measuring teamwork behaviour in the operating theatre. Quality & Safety in Health Care. 2009;**18**(2):104-108. DOI: 10.1136/qshc.2007.024760

[58] Robertson ER, Hadi M, Morgan LJ, et al. Oxford NOTECHS II: A modified theatre team non-technical skills scoring system [published correction appears in PLoS One. 2014;9(6):e100111. Griffin, Damien [corrected to Griffin, Damian]]. PLoS One. 2014;**9**(3):e90320. DOI: 10.1371/journal.pone.0090320

[59] Sharma B, Mishra A, Aggarwal R, Grantcharov TP. Non-technical skills assessment in surgery. Surgical Oncology. 2011;**20**(3):169-177. DOI: 10.1016/j.suronc.2010.10.001

[60] Christian CK, Gustafson ML, Roth EM, et al. A prospective study of patient safety in the operating room. Surgery. 2006;**139**(2):159-173. DOI: 10.1016/j.surg.2005.07.037

[61] Flin R, Patey R. Non-technical skills for anaesthetists: Developing and applying ANTS. Best Practice & Research. Clinical Anaesthesiology. 2011;**25**(2):215-227. DOI: 10.1016/j.bpa.2011.02.005-227

[62] Mitchell L, Flin R, Yule S, Mitchell J, Coutts K, Youngson G. Evaluation of the SPLINTS system for scrub practitioners' non-technical skills. Proceedings of the Human Factors and Ergonomics Society Annual Meeting. 2011;**55**:690-694. DOI: 10.1177/1071181311551143

[63] Fletcher G, Flin R, McGeorge P, Glavin R, Maran N, Anaesthetists PR. Non-technical skills (ANTS): Evaluation of a behavioural marker system. British Journal of Anaesthesia. 2003;**90**(5):580-588. DOI: 10.1093/bja/aeg112

[64] Whittaker G, Abboudi H, Khan MS, Dasgupta P, Ahmed K. Teamwork assessment tools in modern surgical practice: A systematic review. Surgery Research and Practice. 2015;**2015**:494827. DOI: 10.1155/2015/494827

[65] Crossley J, Marriott J, Purdie H, Beard JD. Prospective observational study to evaluate NOTSS (Non-Technical Skills for Surgeons) for assessing trainees' non-technical performance in the operating theatre. The British Journal of Surgery. 2011;**98**(7):1010-1020

[66] Yule S, Flin R, Paterson-Brown S, Maran N, Rowley D. Development of a rating system for surgeons' non-technical skills. Medical Education. 2006;**40**(11):1098-1104

[67] Russ S, Rout S, Sevdalis N, Moorthy K, Darzi A, Vincent C. Do safety checklists improve teamwork and communication in the operating room? A systematic review. Annals of Surgery. 2013;**258**(6):856-871. DOI: 10.1097/SLA.0000000000000206

[68] Lyons VE, Popejoy LL. Meta-analysis of surgical safety checklist effects on teamwork, communication, morbidity, mortality, and safety. Western Journal of Nursing Research. 2014;**36**(2):245-261. DOI: 10.1177/0193945913505782

[69] Nagpal K, Vats A, Ahmed K, et al. A systematic quantitative assessment of risks associated with poor communication in surgical care. Archives of Surgery. 2010;**145**(6):582-588. DOI: 10.1001/archsurg.2010.105

[70] Hull L, Birnbach D, Arora S, Fitzpatrick M, Sevdalis N. Improving surgical ward care: Development and psychometric properties of a global assessment toolkit. Annals of Surgery. 2014;**259**(5):904-909. DOI: 10.1097/SLA.0000000000000451

[71] Rehim SA, DeMoor S, Olmsted R, Dent DL, Parker-Raley J. Tools for assessment of communication skills of hospital action teams: A systematic review. Journal of Surgical Education. 2017;**74**(2):341-351. DOI: 10.1016/j.jsurg.2016.09.008

[72] Chalwin RP, Flabouris A. Utility and assessment of non-technical skills for rapid response systems and medical emergency teams. Internal Medicine Journal. 2013;**43**(9):962-969. DOI: 10.1111/imj.12172

[73] Cooper S, Cant R, Connell C, et al. Measuring teamwork performance: Validity testing of the Team Emergency Assessment Measure (TEAM) with clinical resuscitation teams. Resuscitation. 2016;**101**:97-101. DOI: 10.1016/j.resuscitation.2016.01.026

[74] Osbrun J, Moran L, Musselwhite E. Self-Directed Work Teams: The New American Challenge. Homewood, IL: McGraw-Hill; 1990. pp. 1-26. ISBN 978-1556233418

[75] Katzenbach J, Smith D. The Wisdom of Teams: Creating the High-Performance Organization. 1st ed. Boston: Harvard Business School Press; 1993. pp. 1-26

[76] Chapa OR, Fuller SM, Hernandez LJ, McCray T. Competition versus collaboration in health care teams. Creative Nursing. 2017;**23**(2):97-101. DOI: 10.1891/1078-4535.23.2.97

[77] Paulus P. Groups, teams, and creativity: The creative potential of idea-generating groups. Applied Psychology. 2000;**49**(2):237-262. DOI: 10.1111/1464-0597.00013

[78] Chin R. Examining teamwork and leadership in the fields of public administration, leadership, and management. Team Performance Management. 2015;**21**(3/4):199-216. DOI: 10.1108/TPM-07-2014-0037

[79] Aij KH, Visse M, Widdershoven GA. Lean leadership: An ethnographic study. Leadership in Health Services (Bradford, England). 2015;**28**(2):119-134. DOI: 10.1108/LHS-03-2014-0015

[80] Weberg D. Transformational leadership and staff retention: An evidence review with implications for healthcare systems. Nursing Administration Quarterly. 2010;**34**:246-258. DOI: 10.1097/NAQ.0b013e3181e70298

[81] Menaker R, Bahn RS. How perceived physician leadership behavior affects physician satisfaction. Mayo Clinic Proceedings. 2008;**83**:983-988. DOI: 10.4065/83.9.983

[82] Gowen CR III, Henagan SC, McFadden KL. Knowledge management as a mediator for the efficacy of transformational leadership and quality management initiatives in U.S. health care. Health Care Management Review. 2009;**34**:129-140. DOI: 10.1097/HMR.0b013e31819e9169

[83] Brady Germain P, Cummings GG. The influence of nursing leadership on nurse performance: A systematic literature review. Journal of Nursing Management. 2010;**18**:425-439. DOI: 10.1111/j.1365-2834.2010.01100.x

[84] Stockwell DC, Slonim AD, Pollack MM. Physician team management affects goal achievement in the intensive care unit. Pediatric Critical Care Medicine. 2007;**8**:540-545. DOI: 10.1097/01.PCC.0000288709.15113.8A

[85] Wong CA, Cummings GG. The relationship between nursing leadership and patient outcomes: A systematic review. Journal of Nursing

Management. 2007;**15**:508-521. DOI: 10.1111/j.1365-2834.2007.00723.x

[86] Hix C, McKeon L, Walters S. Clinical nurse leader impact on clinical microsystems outcomes. The Journal of Nursing Administration. 2009;**39**:71-76. DOI: 10.1097/NNA.0b013e318195a612

[87] Horner M. Leadership theory: Past, present and future. Team Performance Management. 1997;**3**(4):270-287. DOI: 10.1108/13527599710195402

[88] Barbuto JE. Scale development and construct clarification of servant leadership. Group & Organization Management. 2006;**31**(3):300-326. DOI: 10.1177/1059601106287091

[89] Spears L. Reflections on Robert K. Greenleaf and servant leadership. Leadership and Organization Development Journal. 1996;**17**(7):33-35. DOI: 10.1108/01437739610148367

[90] Stone AG, Russell RF, Patterson K. Transformational versus servant leadership: A difference in leader focus. Leadership and Organization Development Journal. 2004;**25**(4):349-361. DOI: 10.1108/01437730410538671

[91] Hanse JJ, Harlin U, Jarebrant C, Ulin K, Winkel J. The impact of servant leadership dimensions on leader-member exchange among health care professionals. Journal of Nursing Management. 2016;**24**(2):228-234. DOI: 10.1111/jonm.12304

[92] Aij KH, Rapsaniotis S. Leadership requirements for lean versus servant leadership in health care: A systematic review of the literature. Journal of Healthcare Leadership. 2017;**9**:1-14. DOI: 10.2147/JHL.S120166

[93] Sfantou DF, Laliotis A, Patelarou AE, Sifaki-Pistolla D, Matalliotakis M, Patelarou E. Importance of leadership style towards quality of care measures in healthcare settings: A systematic review. Healthcare (Basel). 2017;**5**(4):73. DOI: 10.3390/healthcare5040073

Chapter 9

Outbreak Management and COVID-19 Pandemic

Vasfiye Bayram Değer

Abstract

Humanity has battled with various epidemics, pandemics and natural disasters throughout history since it began to live in communities, still continuing to do so. In the past, it was very difficult to overcome many of these phenomena both at global and regional level, and even many people were killed. However, during the plagues, countries attempted to develop a number of strategies, tactics and methods within the scope of combating the epidemic. At this point, these struggles, measures and actions have facilitated prevention and spread of outbreaks, and sometimes they have not been sufficiently efficacious. On the other hand, struggles with epidemics, pandemics and natural disasters, which deeply affect all segments of the society in terms of social, cultural and economic aspects as well as mental and physical health, have been inherited to the present day, becoming a vast accumulation of practices to be re-applied in possible disasters humanity will face. The main point lies in the fact that here is that the struggles fought in traditional societies and modern societies have different characteristics. Especially in those traditional societies where medicine and technology are underdeveloped, the struggles carried out within uncertain constraints have caused pandemics and epidemics to last longer. The modern society we live in today, on the other hand, is on the verge of several risks and threats unlike traditional societies. When we consider the modern society within the risk society approaches, the present risks should also be thoroughly discussed. In this context, epidemics, which are a type of natural disaster, and the methods of combating them should be investigated within the framework of risk and crisis management due to the risks in modern society.

Keywords: outbreak management, risk management process, outbreak

1. Introduction

Considering the history of outbreaks as a biological phenomenon, it is obvious that they are as old as human history. The most fundamental aspect of this interpretation lies in the acceptance that microorganisms that cause diseases are also much older than human history. The microorganisms, which are the main source of outbreaks that cause the mass casualties, have not been recognized for a long time because they are too small to be discovered. However, it is possible to evaluate the lifestyles in traditional societies as one of the involving factors in the lack of knowledge about the diseases [1]. Since the risk of contracting any epidemic disease was low in traditional society periods when there was no sedentary life and people relied their lives on hunting and gathering, it was nearly impossible to know about these diseases. On the other hand, it was not possible for the outbreak to be lasting for a

IntechOpen

long time because the persistence of the disease among people required the need for a large human population. However, with the subsequent transition to sedentary life, many contributing factors have also emerged, causing the diseases to spread easily. Consequently, awareness about outbreaks has increased and the names and systematic of outbreaks in history have started to be discussed [2].

The outbreaks are classified and termed according to their scientific structure and characteristics, spreading areas and the size of population they affect. At this point, an outbreak is divided into three categories as endemic, epidemic and pandemic. In ancient Greek, the word "en" means inside and the word "demos" means people. Derived from the combination of these two words, "endemics" is the term used to describe a disease that has always existed in a given population and can survive in a given population without external influence. The word "epidemic" is derived from the combination of the ancient Greek words "epi" meaning on or over and "demos" meaning people. In order for a disease to be defined as an epidemics, it must be prevalent in a certain human population within a certain period of time and have a pervasive effect more than expected compared to previous experiences. Finally, the term pandemic is derived from the ancient Greek word "pan" meaning all and "demos" meaning people. Unlike endemics and epidemics, pandemics refers to the type of disease that spreads over a continent or even the entire world [3].

The typical course of the disease in a pandemic with a global impact is explained as follows: The infection spreads to healthy people in a short time. It is acute and severe in its course. Those who contract the infection either die or recover completely in a short time. Finally, the survivors can develop long-term or lifelong immunity to the infection. Indicating a typical cycle of an infectious outbreak, the above steps have caused numerous casualties throughout history and left indelible marks in the areas they affected. These infections emerged as epidemics, some of which lasted for a short time or a long time, but each time caused many deaths, and humanity tried to take measures against and overcome them. On the other hand, the outbreaks have led to momentous economic, administrative, social and political changes in societies other than casualties [4]. Given the effects of past and recent epidemics on individuals and society, it is seen that epidemics are not only biological phenomena that threaten the public health but also diseases that trigger changes and transformations in all areas of life [5].

The outbreaks whose prevalence and recognition increased as humanity started to live in large settlements with crowded groups caused millions of people to suffer and lose their lives throughout history. Regarding epidemics, Diamond stated that the disease has an exclusive cycle in itself [6]. According to Diamond, epidemics are defined as the type of disease during which the sick people infect the people around them rather than individual chronic cases and the majority of the population contracts the disease in a very short time. In addition, another major characteristics of epidemics is that they progress acutely and ultimately result in death or recovery in a short time [6]. Due to their inherent characteristics, epidemics have culminated in great political, social, economic, cultural and psychological devastation in the societies where they emerged. The literature review shows that approximately three major plagues, seven cholera outbreaks and more than 10 influenza pandemics have occurred since ancient times, affecting the entire social order. Epidemic outbreaks of smallpox, yellow fever and malaria have had almost as devastating effects as the pandemics aforementioned [7].

When the diseases that broke out in the past are examined, as stated above, people and their established systems were affected in terms of politics, socio-economic life, and mental health. The epidemics have exerted great impacts that even changed the course of battles and led to changes in power and order. When the battles in history are examined, it is seen that the epidemics changed the outcome of many wars, caused the collapse of empires, and even states used these epidemics as a martial strategy [6]. As a matter of fact, the Peleponnesian wars are one of the most popular examples showing that epidemic diseases affect the results of wars [8]. Thucydides [9] explained the severity of the disease that plagued the Peloponnesian Wars and changed the course of the war in favor of the Athenians with the following words: "The disease was so severe that no one knew what would happen, and respect for everything divine and venerable was lost." As a matter of fact, even Pericles, the honourable statesman of the Athenians, died during the war due to the epidemic. Besides affecting the results of the wars, epidemics also affected the military organization and the urban planning and castle architecture [10]. In the Roman Empire, for example, the duty of the military medical troop is commissioned not only to treat the soldiers wounded in wars, but also prevent the spread of epidemics. However, it is estimated that epidemics caused significant problems in economic and commercial life, increased the cost of goods and services, social confusion and chaos caused by mass migration. In addition, the death rates caused by the epidemics experienced in the past were quite high compared to those by others. The major reasons for can be listed as inability to make an early diagnosis of the disease and determine the source as well as lack of means to prevent the transmission routes, and lastly primitivity of technology [5].

When the epidemics in history are examined, one of the epidemics that claims mass deaths other than the bubonic plague and cholera and continues to do so even today is the influenza epidemic. It is the most common acute and febrile respiratory disease in its broadest meaning [1]. The disease, also called as influenza in medicine, is caused by A, B and C type viruses. Its course can be mild and uncertain, and in some cases, complications that cause death may occur. The worst complication is pneumonia caused by the infection affecting the lungs. It is known that the influenza is an infectious disease whch have caused more than 10 pandemics most of which originated from China since ancient times. Unlike diseases such as plague, cholera, smallpox, measles or malaria, the influenza is not a viral disease that causes death or deformities in the human body in a short time. The most prominant characteristics of influenza is that the virus causing the infection can be mutated continuously and the treatment of the disease can vary in parallel with its changed state. Therefore, it may take long time to provide treatment against the influenza caused by viruses not recognized by the body [1].

The first known influenza epidemic in history struck Italy and France in 1173. The epidemic in 1580 can be considered as the first one in history. It occurred in Asia and spread to Africa, Europe and the U.S. Later, another epidemic that started in Russia between 1729–1733 pervaded the whole Europe. Then, in 1781, another influenza pandemic, started in China and spread throughout Europe and the U.S. Moreover, with the development of transportation and communication networks, influenza epidemics have become more and more prevalent. As a matter of fact, three more pandemics occurred between 1830–1831, in 1883 and 1889–1890. The most remarkable of these pandemics broke out in Russia between 1889–1890, then spread to Europe and was called as the Russian Flu [11]. By 1918, another epidemic called Swine Flu occurred in three waves, again causing the deaths of millions of people. During the epidemic encountered in this period, it was found that more than four million people died in the U.S. alone [1]. In the subsequent periods, three more influenza pandemics originated from China and spread to different continents. During the Asian Flu in 1957 and the Hong Kong Flu pandemics in 1968–1970, more than one million people died worldwide. These pandemics were followed by SARS (Severe Acute Respiratory Syndrome) in 2003, Swine Flu in 2009–2010, MERS (Middle East Respiratory Syndrome) in 2015 and lastly 2020 COVID-19 Pandemic caused by Coronavirus. When the vast epidemics and pandemics in the history are examined, it is obvious that the plague, cholera and influenza outbreaks generally emerge as pandemics. On the other hand, those epidemics and endemics that were effective in the region where they originated have reached dimensions that could threaten human health and have caused mass deaths. The most common of these diseases include smallpox, measles, mumps, typhoid, typhus, HIV/AIDS, malaria, fever and EBOLA [5].

By definition, the concept of risk management does not necessarily mean preventing the risk completely, but rather refers to approaching the problems systematically and carefully as well as preventing unnecessary losses through careful management of the risks that are decided to take [12].

The important points in risk management involve recognizing the risk clearly enough, diagnosing it correctly, seeking ways to eliminate the risk, and transferring the risk by minimizing it. In this context, in order to overcome the Covid-19 pandemic process with the least damage, the precautions must be absolutely examined in view of risk management. In addition, crisis management, which will maximize the success of risk management, should not be undermined. Therefore, the definition of crisis crisis refers to a difficult moment or a certain period of depression in the life of a person, an organization or a society. In this respect, when the crisis is evaluated, its uncertainty includes the possibility of harm and risk within itself [13]. Hence, considering the relationship between risk management and crisis management, it is necessary to state that the risk precedes the crisis and so does the risk management. However, it is also apparent that there is a relational cycle between risk management and crisis management processes in terms of epidemic management. If more risk factors identified in the epidemic management process are reduced and the probabilities are predicted better, then they can be used more often in determining future projections along with more precautions taken to reduce risks and develop appropriate policies, which ultimately contributes to more effective crisis management from the moment the crises occur [4].

In this context, successful implementation of the activities conducted to battle against the epidemic around the world and in Turkey, it is imperative that the course of the epidemic be evaluated in terms of risk and crisis management to achieve lasting and effective results. However, taking the historical background and past experiences into account while planning risk and crisis management will be one of the most crucial strategies.

In general, the concept of risk means something that includes uncertainties in itself. The risk exists if statistics of probable distributions can be calculated for the outcomes of any given situation while uncertainty exists if there is no common attitude towards such a situation. Due to uncertain characteristics of risk, failure to make statistical inferences about a subject, and the uncertainty of repeatable risk situations even if they are made, cause a lack of foresight in terms of decision-making and planning. Therefore, it is necessary to state that any uncertainty is one of the important points to be evaluated within the scope of risk management. In classical risk analysis approaches, it is stated that decision-makers should evaluate the situation with a holistic perspective, taking the uncertainty into the scope of the analysis according to possible future results [14]. In order to determine the risk factors in risk analysis, a pre-risk scanning system should be established at first. The activities carried out in the screening system also require an effective crisis management since the goal in risk management is not to eliminate the risk, but to overcome the crisis by minimizing the damage in the event of a possible crisis [15]. Hence, it is necessary to activate the process of crisis management in determining the ways to be followed in risk analysis. As a matter of fact, the steps in the scanning system that are determined in analyzing the risks in risk analysis approaches are defined in relation to the crisis and crisis management. According to Özer [16]; the steps determined in the scanning system that makes risk analysis possible are presented below;

Problem Management: The solution of the existing problem is evaluated as a type of problem that will affect those at risk. In this step, the negative effects of the problem are tried to be reduced. In this respect, the problems must be classified into short and long term effective categories. Since some problems may trigger crises in the long or short term, crisis screening should also be done for them.

Risk Evaluation: In this step, weaknesses that may cause a crisis are determined by defining risk factors. Therefore, a number of measures must be taken to eliminate weaknesses before possible crisis situations are identified.

Relations with Groups at Risk: In risk situations, the groups that will be most affected by the threats of this risk must be determined and contacted. Communication with these groups will be most effective and useful in times of crisis.

By raising awareness before the crisis, the panic situations that will occur during the crisis and the new risks and crises to be created by these situations will be prevented. The risk screening system formed by determining the steps above will render the risk determination process more concrete and planned. In the implementation of the risk screening system, a successful risk management process must be performed by following the steps of defining, measuring, judging and evaluating the risk and finally analysing it. In the risk management process, it is targeted at the basic identification, control and recording of the threats and opportunities, minimizing the risks, maximizing the gains, preventing and reducing the losses, optimizing the gains, managing the crisis effectively and finally reaching at the maximum management capacity [16]. If we schematically express the risk management process under general headings in line with the steps listed above, the following steps will appear.

In line with the steps given in **Figure 1** regarding the risk management process, in case of an infectious outbreak, the current risk situation must fit be identified. Elimination of the uncertainty about the existence of the risk situation is a priority in order to determine the next steps to be followed. When making risk evaluation after the situation is identified, the harming potential (impact) of the disease, the

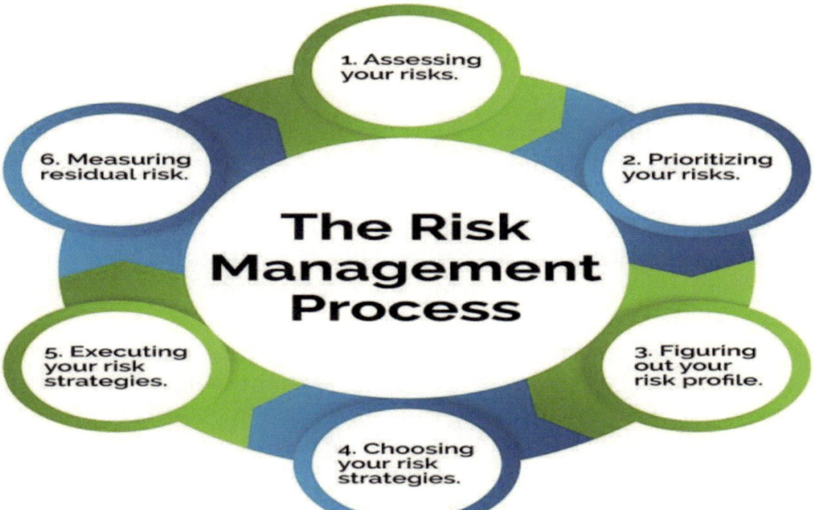

Figure 1.
Risk Management Process (https://www.mha-it.com/2020/01/29/risk-management/).

rate of exposure to the agent in the society and the susceptibility of the society must be taken into account. However, a number of questions arise in the following: Who are the population or groups at risk? What is the level of risk evaluation (local, regional, national etc.)? Who are the people who will carry out the risk evaluation phase? and What is the time frame specified in the risk evaluation?. Seeking reasonable answers to these well-defined questions during the epidemic will enable the risk evaluation phase to be carried out more systematically [17].

Risk control and precautionary analysis following the risk evaluation phase are of vital importance for risk management since the tools and precise strategies that reduce, inhibit or eliminate the risk are determined at this step [18]. At this point, it is necessary to identify a number of methods in line with the data obtained from the epidemics in the past. However, the formation of a team of experts in the field considering the essence of the decisions to be taken is important in determining the strategy and tactics to be practised. Otherwise, that will bring about new risk situations. Another point to be mentioned about this step is to ensure that all segments of the society are aware of the determined methods and strategies through means of modern information technologies. In this process, the mental health of the society must be thoroughly monitored while the existing bad conditions should be improved as much as possible and the hopeful message that no individual in the society is alone and this challenging process will be overcome together should be communicated. These steps requiring an effective use of mass media must also be managed accurately and in a controlled manner.

The tools and methods that ensure risk control are identified in the third step by considering all uncertain, probable and certain situations, and the necessary decisions are taken to move to the next step [19]. These decisions are taken by the administrators who are in appropriate positions and the process of making controlled decisions is initiated by analyzing all costs and benefits [16].

In the fourth step of implementing the decisions taken, the strategies determined and developed by using time and resources are started to be practised. In order to achieve that, a good communication between decision-makers and the risk group must be established beforehand. In the previous stages, it is necessary to convey the decisions taken to those in the risk group properly, to express the expected attitudes from the risk group and to ensure the maximum participation of everyone in the risk group since this step will ensure elimination of the threats, reduction of the effects of the threats or minimization of the number of people affected by the threats. Therefore, the actions to be performed require a high level of coordination and harmony [5].

After the successful implementation of the decisions, the next action is to monitor thecourse of the event. In the process of monitoring the event, problems must be identified and eliminated if possible while the people in the risk group should be encouraged to abide by the decisions and the control efficiency of the process must be ensured for the continuity of the process [18]. Then, the same process must be repeated by making a risk evaluation for new situations that occur after the decisions made [18].

In order to go through a successful risk management process, the aforementioned five steps must be fulfilled in accordance with the requirements. In addition, individuals or groups that play an active role in the risk management process should pay attention to some factors including "avoiding unnecessary risk, taking risk decisions at the appropriate level, accepting risk when the benefits are superior to the costs" [19].

While evaluating epidemics in terms of risk, crisis, risk and crisis management, it can be said that the risk during such outbreaks is generally a combination of the possibility of an infectious disease to trigger an epidemic and its impact size [17].

On the other hand, a crisis refers to an unpredictable, unexpected and unusual situation that occurs abruptly [20]. From this point of view, it should be stated that epidemics that cannot be identifed by the health community also create a crisis situation. In addition, the risk may also vary depending on the conditions of the country/region, political landscape, perceived risk and interest of the media and society. On the other hand, crisis situations are also shaped by the perceptions of the masses. The extent of the crisis is affected by the life experiences of the society where it emerges in view of the perception of the threat it created. Therefore, probabilities such as the emergence of crises, their impact, and the groups they will affect should be taken into serious consideration when making a risk evaluation. The main purpose of risk evaluation within the scope of combating unknown/unidentified epidemics is to initiate emergency interventions, constrict the epidemic with a specific treatment and non-pharmaceutical public health measures specifically for the disease that is not eliminated by a vaccine when the disease is first encountered, and mitigate its impact. In this context, performing a risk analysis/evaluation refers to a process that is started by identifying the event and continues until it is taken under control [17]. Therefore, the steps of the risk scanning system in the aforementioned risk analysis approach should be carried out systematically in the risk management process. In addition, risk assessment carried out with the screening steps within the scope of risk analysis should be carried out with an interdisciplinary approach by experts in the field and with the participation of the society in the process. On the other hand, the crisis and crisis management issues should not be ignored while performing risk analysis and evaluation. Identification of threatening issues should also be considered in the context of crisis management since there is a high probability of crises to occur in situations where risks exist [5].

The questions to be answered in order to determine the crisis possibilities in risk management and to terminate the process successfully care as follows [13]:

- What is the critical level of the situation?
- What is the worst thing that could take place?
- What is the main factor of this chaos?
- What are the alternative solutions?
- Which groups/persons will be affected by this situation at the most?
- What is the expected attitude of the groups that will be affected by this situation during the crisis?
- What is the fundamental strategy to be put into action in case of an expected crisis?
- Who should take action throughout the process?

Strategic methods and tactics determined in line with the answers given to these questions should be applied in relation to risk and crisis management.

One of the issues strongly emphasized in evaluating risks and crises in terms of outbreaks is sharing the results of the risk analysis, in other words, proper communication of the identified risk. The risk must be interpreted and shared with the parties at every stage of the evaluation. Communicating or sharing the risk with appropriate language will not only help the public to prepare for the measures to be taken and increase participation, but also guide the preparation of protocols for laboratory-based test development, diagnosis, monitoring and treatment [4].

Risk, crisis management and evaluation processes are defined as a combined process of three-components in which up-to-date information is collected, evaluated and recorded on a continuous and regular basis to manage an acute public health issue [5]. It is possible to categorize these components into three gorups: threat, exposure and contextual evaluation. In the threat evaluation of an epidemic, answers to the following questions are sought;

- Does the epidemic virus cause disease in humans?
- What are the clinical findings of the disease?
- What characteristics of humans do make them vulnerable to the disease?
- Is it a formerly encountered disease?
- Are there any special factors for the spread of the disease?
- Which findings can help us in its diagnosis?
- Is there an effective treatment method for the disease?

Secondly, answers to the following questions are sought in the exposure evaluation:

- How many people get sick?
- What are the ways of transmission?,
- What is the level of contagiousness of the disease?
- What kind of symptoms does the disease cause on the patient?
- Can the symptoms of the disease cause permanent or temporary health damage?

Finally, answers to the following questions are sought in the contextual evaluation;

- What kind of effects does the disease have at local, regional, national and global level?
- What is the susceptibility of the society to the disease in the local environment?
- How does the healthy and cultural behavior of individuals in the society affect the course of the disease?

In the event of an epidemic, the answers sought to the questions listed above and the answers given to these questions will make it possible to make a successful risk and crisis management evaluation about the disease. Another important issue at this point is to be able to adapt past experiences to today's conditions by learning from past experiences and knowledge, whether or not the disease that caused the epidemic has the same characteristics as in the previous period. As a matter of fact, making these adaptations is one of the main factors that will enable us to carry out risk and crisis management effectively [5].

The COVID-19 outbreak that started in Wuhan, China; On March 11, 2020, more than 118,000 cases in 114 countries reached 4291 deaths and were approved by the World Health Organization (WHO) as a pandemic [21]. Since WHO proclamation of COVID-19 as a pandemic, the global spread rate has increased and the spread in the society persists in many countries. Updated number of cases and an interactive map highlighting confirmed cases worldwide are available on the websites of the World Health Organization and the European Center for Disease Prevention and Control [22].

Infection is mainly transmitted through droplets. It is generally reported that the incubation period is between 2–14 days and the average incubation period is 4.8 days. The contagious period of COVID-19 is not exactly known. It is thought that it starts a couple of days before symptomatic period and ends up with fading of symptoms [23]. The whole society is vulnerable to COVID-19. Healthcare professionals are the most risky occupational group in terms of encountering the infectious agent. Men, people over the age of 50, those with comorbidities (hypertension, cardicac disease, diabetes mellitus, malignancy, COPD, renal failure, etc.), seasonal agricultural workers and those living in nursing and rehabilitation centres, schools, barracks, detention houses and immigration camps are among vulnerable groups in terms of COVID-19. The clinical indicators of infection range from non-mild symptoms to severe pneumonia with organic functional damage. Common symptoms include fever, cough, dyspnoea and myalgia. Symptoms such as sore throat, chest pain, hemoptysis, conjunctival congestion, nausea and vomiting, headache, runny nose, painful muscles and joints, extreme weakness, loss of smell and taste, and diarrhea can also be seen [24]. The first COVID-19 diagnosis in Turkey was made on March 11, 2020, and some precautionary actions were taken to prevent the spread of the disease and to treat patients. In line with the epidemic plan, a multi-sectoral approach has been applied and preventive measures have been put into practice that address the society as a whole. During this process, pandemic action decisions started to be implemented in Family Health Units. The administrational decisions register that is approved by every physician working at the Family Healthcare Centre included the measures to be taken during the pandemic process and the changes to be made in FHC's operation in written form [24]. There is no vaccine or medicine yet to protect against COVID-19. The best way to prevent the infection is to avoid exposure to the virüs [25].

2. Global overview

In China, efforts to prevent spread of COVID-19 have been used the basic principles that include identifying and isolating infectious sources and cutting off transmission routes. As of January 31, 2020, about 12,000 cases were confirmed and 18,000 cases were suspected in China. Studies have reported that the spread of COVID-19 is relatively rapid and reached to many other countries after its outbreak in China. On January 31, 2020, 213 cases of deaths were reported worldwide. As of the same date, confirmed cases have been reported in the following 19 countries outside China: Australia (n = 9), Canada (n = 3), Cambodia (n = 1), France (n = 6),

Finland (n = 1), Germany (n = 5), India (n = 1), Italy (n = 2), Japan (n = 14), Nepal (n = 1), Malaysia (n = 8), the Philippines (n = 1), Republic of Korea (n = 11), Singapore (n = 13), Sri Lanka (n = 1), Thailand (n = 14), United States of America (n = 6), United Arab Emirates (n = 4) and Vietnam (n = 5) [26, 27].

The disease gradually spread all over the world and the epicenter of the pandemic subsequently shifted from Wuhan in China to Europe and the USA. The infection has a very dynamic structure spreading rapidly. The number of confirmed cases varies due to differences in epidemiological surveillance and diagnostic capacities across countries. Since a reliable treatment method has not yet been devised for this type of virus, controlling the rate of spread requires effective planning of healthcare infrastructure and services. Therefore, the estimation of the total confirmed cases and possible new cases in the future is vital for directing the demand to the healthcare system and managing the pandemic [28].

Italy is the first country in Europe to be seriously challenged by a large number of deaths from COVID-19, followed by Spain, France, Germany and the United Kingdom. European countries have taken measures such as flight restrictions, closing down borders, cafes and restaurants, and suspending education to prevent the spread of the disease. The UK and the Netherlands took a ethically different and ominous approach targeting at herd immunity. However, even these two countries eventually had to resort to some measures and restrictions [29]. In the USA, the first COVID-19 case was reported in Washington State on January 15, 2020 [30]. On January 20, state and local health departments in the United States initiated monitoring of all people thought to have had close contact with people infected with COVID-19. The purpose of these efforts is to ensure rapid evaluation and care of patients, limit further transmission and better understand underlying risk factors. A number of measures such as active symptom monitoring consisting of daily phone calls, texting or face-to-face conversations about fever or other symptoms during the 14 days following the last known exposure to a COVID-19 confirmed person, were conducted by local health organizations. In addition, specific guidelines for health services (infection control and prevention, laboratory testing, environmental cleaning, worker safety and international travel etc.) including patient management have been developed and published online. These guides are updated as we learn more. US public health authorities still continue to study on clarification of virus incubation period and duration with implications for quarantine time and other mitigation measures, the relative importance of various modes of transmission (understanding these modes of transmission has major implications for infection control and prevention, including the use of personal protective equipment, determination of the severity and fatality rate of COVD-19 in the US health system, as well as more detailed description of the infection spectrum and risk factors, identification of the role of asymptomatic infection in ongoing transmission; and to assist in the development of vaccines and therapeutic interventions and finally evaluating the immunological response to infection. As of June 27, 2020, the total number of diagnosed cases worldwide reached 9.9 million. The number of people who lost their lives was nearly 500,000. The United States was the country with the highest number of cases (n = 2.5 million), followed by Brazil (n = 1,280,000), Russia (n = 627,000) and India (n = 510,000) respectively. The highest number in Europe was seen in the UK with 310,000 cases. Other countries in Europe with a high number of cases were Spain (n = 295,000), Italy (n = 240,000) and Germany (n = 195,000) respectively. Considering the number of casulties, the United States ranked as the first country with 127,000 deaths. Other countries with a high number of deaths are Brazil (n = 56,000), United Kingdom (n = 43,000), Italy (n = 34,000) and France (n = 29,000) respectively [24, 31].

DOI: http://dx.doi.org/10.5772/intechopen.96335

3. Overview of Turkey

The first detected cases of Covid-19 were announced on 11 March 2020 by the Ministry of Health in Turkey and the first death case due to the virus took place on 15 March, 2020. The Ministry of Health also announced that coronavirus cases were confirmed all over Turkey on 1 April, 2020. As of June 27, 2020 the number of people infected with the coronavirus in Turkey was 190,000 while the number of those who lost their lives due to virus was about 5,000. On this date, Turkey outnumbered China where the first cases were seen and ranked 12th after Germany while ranking as 17th among 185 countries in view of death cases [24].

4. COVID-19 outbrak management in Turkey

The Ministry of Health established an Operational Center on January 10, 2020 against possible risks after the COVID-19 outbreak started in China, and urgently formed the Scientific Committee, which plays a critical role in outbreak management. COVID-19 outbreak management is carried out under the coordination of the Ministry of Health and in cooperation with the sectors within the framework of the "Pandemic Influenza National Preparation Plan", taking into account the recommendations of the Scientific Advisory Board. The impact of the COVID-19 measures taken by central institutions and organizations is increased by the city-specific evaluations made by the "Provincial Pandemic Committees". During the outbreak period, required measures are taken and implemented for the infection chain specific to COVID-19 within the scope of public health management. These measures can be classified as source-oriented measures (detection and notification of infected persons, isolation and treatment of the patient, filiation, screening studies, examination and follow-up of contacts, quarantine practices, health education), measures for the route of transmission (social distance, hand hygiene, respiratory hygiene, surface cleaning, disinfection, frequent ventilation of indoor environments, improvement of indoor air quality, use of appropriate personal protective equipment and health education in line with the risks when necessary, and measures for the host (health education, adequate and balanced nutrition, sufficient and regular sleep, physical exercise, cessation of smoking, etc.), reducing the possibility of exposure to the agent (limiting collective activities in the streets, flexible working/working from home, reducing contact time, shortening the shifts and organizing rest intervals, etc.) and early diagnosis and treatment of cases [32].

Community-level measures have also been initiated while finding and monitoring the cases and their contacts. When starting or ending a measure against the community, factors such as costs, social problems and "precautionary burnout" in the society are taken into account, ensuring that they will not cause an increase in cases again. Different communication strategies are used effectively to ensure social participation since the compliance of the society with the measures is an important factor in outbreak control. Compliance with different measures is monitored by qualitative and quantitative methods, and new measures are taken against decreased compliance and burnout over time. The size of the measures may differ according to the risk level and local measures may be required by surveillance data. In addition to the "Provincial Pandemic Plan", "number of new cases, incidence and cumulative incidence rate, number of cases and distribution of incidence by district, age group, gender, vulnerable groups etc., number of cases healing daily, and mortality rates" are used in order to evaluate the COVID-19 outbreak at the provincial level [24].

An effective surveillance system should be implemented in order to make evidence-based decisions in outbreak management at national and provincial/ district level. Coordination between central and provincial organizations should be carried out at the highest level in outbreak control and prevention procedures by sharing data analysis and evaluations at the provincial/district level with the teams involved in the data collection process [24].

5. Primary COVID-19 outbreak management in Turkey.

In the light of this information, the most critical measure to be taken during the pandemic process is usage of personal protective equipment (PPE) by the whole society, especially healthcare workers. In order to prevent the coexistence of healthy people and possible COVID-19 cases and transmission routes at the first contact places of the health system, WHO's screening and triage recommendations for COVID-19 should be followed [33]. For this reason, Family Health Unit (FHU) employees were made to wear PPE (mask, gloves, visor or goggles, aprons) and every patient admitted was obliged to wear a mask. A triage unit has been created at the entrance of FHU. By measuring the fever of each patient and questioning his/ her history (fever, cough, breathing difficulty, contact and travel history), possible COVID-19 cases were tried to be diagnosed by the assistant health personnel working here (nurse, midwife, paramedics). Suspected cases were evaluated by taking them to the isolation unit at the entrance of the FHU and thus the possible contamination risk was reduced. Patients deemed at risk were referred to a higher level health institution by contacting the Provincial Health Directorate. The patients who were not deemed to be at risk were admitted in a certain order in accordance with social distance rules and the size of the FHU waiting rooms. Hand disinfectants were available in FHU entrances and exit and waiting rooms. Procedures for FHU hygiene were restructured in accordance with the directives of the Ministry of Health [33].

In Family Health Units where primary health care services are provided, preventive health services are most frequently resorted for medical procedures such as having an examination, prescribing medication, getting an injection, dressing and various health reports. People can access all these services by applying to their registered family physician, patients were primarily directed to family health centers by the Ministry of Health in order to reduce crowding that may occur in secondary and tertiary healthcare providers during the pandemic process, and some regulations were remade for FHU applications [33].

Treatments and preventive health services are provided together in primary health care institutions. Preventive health services include primary, secondary and tertiary prevention [33]. Primary prevention involves the procedures performed to prevent or eliminate the cause of any health problem before it emerges in the individual or society. Secondary prevention includes the measures taken to identify a health problem in a person or community at an earlier stage. In this way, treatment becomes easier, thereby its spread is prevented and its impact is decreased in the long term [34]. Considering how simple but effective measures such as quitting smoking and avoiding obesity can prevent many diseases and save lives, the importance of especially primary preventive health services can be understood better. During the COVID-19 pandemic, primary and secondary prevention methods have been effectively used. The precautions taken to avoid contact with the virus and the early diagnosis and isolation of the contacts from the environment played a leading role in attenuating the impact of COVID-19 pandemic. Many health policies have been created to prevent this contact. In our country, in order to control the epidemic, to identify the first source, and to monitor and isolate the contacts, filiation was enforced under the leadership of Provincial Health Directorates/Community Health Centers in accordance with the rules determined by the Ministry of Health. During the pandemic process, family physicians also took an active role in the filiation. Persons at risk were monitored by the family physicians and/or family health workers in line with the criteria set by the Ministry of Health. A person with confirmed or suspected COVID-19 and others who had close contact without taking protective measures against droplets were quarantined for 14 days after their last contact. Those whose tests were negative were quarantined for 14 days. Those whose tests were positive were quarantined for 14 days after 4 days without symptoms. Those who completed military service were quarantined for 14 days after they returned home. Those who were abroad and returned home were quarantined for 14 days. All these people were questioned by phone especially in terms of fever and respiratory symptoms, and informed about the quarantine conditions and closely monitored [33].

As a result, the COVID-19 pandemic has deeply affected our lives in our country as well as all over the world and showed that we need to rearrange our life norms. It is inevitable that such kind of epidemics will recur in the globalizing world. Therefore, social awareness and protective measures are essential. İn the Covid-19 outbreak everyone should be vigilant until the last case is healed, and precautions taken in family health centers, which are the front line of health services, should continue to be implemented. Preventive health services should be constantly supported, and risky/possible cases should be monitored and filiation should be continued [33].

The COVID-19 pandemic had severe health and economic consequences both in the world and in our country. An effective treatment and vaccine for the infection has not yet been found. The best intervention that could be done to reduce the contagiousness of the disease is to maintain social distance, comply with hygiene rules and wear a mask. Community immunity is another way to control pandemics. In short, it is a way of protecting individuals indirectly from an epidemic to develop immunity in the majority of the population. When it is desired to ensure community immunity by reducing protective measures, the number of cases and deaths will be increased. On the other hand, when it is desired to maintain strict protective measures until the vaccine is produced, it will take time to be widely implemented in the world. Political decision-makers should work in coordination with academia, relevant governmental institutions and non-governmental organizations in order to evaluate the psychological, sociological and economic effects of maintaining all the measures in the society and to make the best decision within the possible benefit/loss relationship.

An outbreak management, as stated by İnandı and et al. [16], should be addressed as follows. Considering the differences in dynamics and intervention methods, the outbreak can be examined in five phases:

Initial Phase: During this period, sporadic and importing cases emerge. Cases are localized at first and transmission is slow. Then clusters of cases begin to appear.

Peak Phase: It is the period when there is widespread human-to-human transmission in the community and the outbreak curve begins to rise. In this period, the reproduction number-defined as R0 (the average number of new patients that a patient can infect the disease in a fully susceptible society) is greater than 1 and the number of patients in the community gradually grows. If the contagiousness of the agent is high, the number of sick people may increase in a very short time and constrain the capacity of health systems. During the outbreak, as some people get sick, the susceptible population will decrease. R0 changes and this new reproduction number is called as the effective reproduction number - Re [35]. During the peak period, the concept of "the number of cases increasing exponentially" is also an important concept. If no precautions are taken, the number of people affected in the epidemic increases rapidly and exponentially, as each sick patient infects the disease to new people. In this phase, the number of days to double the cases is short.

Plateau Phase: The peak is followed by the plateau phase, in which the rate of increase in cases decreases. During this period, the number of patients detected daily is high while there is no significant increase compared to the previous days. The outbreak curve forms a near-straight line. The Re value is about 1.

Bottom Phase: There is a continuous decrease in the number of new cases. Although Re is below 1, it is still close to 1 and the control of the disease has not been fully achieved yet.

Control Phase: It is the phase where the number of new patients is substantially reduced and a flat course is seen because the outbreak is under control or people in the community have recovered to a large extent. At this stage, Re value is below 1 and gradually decreases. If the disease inherits immunity, the longer the time in the epidemic increases, the less susceptible people are. The presence of the vaccine and its administration to susceptible people are important in controlling the epidemic. Person-to-person transmission can be avoided by reducing the number of susceptible people through vaccination (community immunity), but this is unlikely for COVID-19 since there is currently no effective vaccine available.

6. Indicators that can be used for decision-makers to evaluate risks and intervention according to the stages of the outbreaks

As in the chain of infection in all infectious diseases, the agent in COVID-19 (source) arises as a result of the interaction between the transmission route and the host. Breaking this chain through various interventions will provide the opportunity to control the epidemic at first and then interrupt it. These interventions range from efforts that focus on limiting the disease in a specific region (suppression) to reducing the social effects of the epidemic (impact reduction), and this variability also reveals the differences in crisis management strategies of the countries [36]. In this period when there is no progress in vaccination and treatment, it is aimed to minimize the "impact" that will arise by evaluating the interventions aimed at lessening social exposure together with the risk. Case-specific decision matrices are used in scoring this impact and risk evaluations are made by crossing the risk elements and the availability of intervention tools. An example of this type of risk scoring has been used by the World Health Organization to evaluate sporting events and religious activities in terms of COVID risk [17].

İnandı (2020) and hıs frıends the risk factors and intervention opportunities specific to the upward and downward stages of the epidemic prepared by reviewing the guidelines and recommendations of the Ministry of Health, national and international organizations are grouped below [17]. Here, the risks and intervention tools that decision makers should consider in their own provinces are pointed out. It is possible to duplicate the indicators presented in this table. To do this, the "question generator" approach described in the risk assessment section of the article can be used. When appropriate questions are asked according to the phase of the outbreak, relevant indicators can be created as shown in the table. For example, the following questions can be asked to determine the indicators for populational characteristics:

- What is the rate of the high risk age group in terms of infection in your province?

- Since it increases the risk of contact in our city, what are the places/districts where the population density is high?

DOI: http://dx.doi.org/10.5772/intechopen.96335

Intervention possibilities according to the phases of the outbreak are also listed below. Accordingly, for example, if it is concluded that the risk has been evaluated during the bottom phase and the risk is reduced, appropriate interventions can be selected and implemented gradually in health services at community and individual level.

7. Examination of risk factors and intervention opportunities according to different phases of the outbreak

7.1 Peak/Plateau

7.1.1 Risk factors

- Population and geographical features
- Populational characteristics (population aged 60 and over, population density)
- Presence of places where people live together such as prison, military barracks, nursing home, etc.
- Multiplicity of disadvantaged groups (such as immigrants, poor groups)
- Distribution of the population by educational, income and social security status, existence of regions where inequalities are highly concentrated
- Features of working and economic life (Heavy industry, informal working conditions, child labor, seasonal work, high number of touristical businesses, etc.)
- Neighborhoods of the city (infectional status of neighboring provinces or bordering with the country affected by the outbreak)
- Business of travelling (airports, presence of an airport with international flights, road mobility)

7.1.2 Morbidity and Mortality Criteria

- Status of the general health indicators of the province (maternal and infant deaths, vaccination rates, etc.)
- The prevalence of the groups susceptible to coronavirus (such as DM, CHD, COPD, HT)
- Basic epidemiological information regarding the outbreak and the availability of this information (distribution by age, location, specific groups, detailed data on test practices, contacts, treatment, isolation and quarantine processes)
- Existence of a region with a cluster of cases
- Mortality criteria (distribution of deaths by age and gender, rates specific to disease groups/risk factors, case fatality rate)
- Completeness, accuracy and transparency of all health records, especially the death registration system

- Health Services
- Pre-epidemic status of primary health care services (population per family physician, number of nurses)
- Pre-epidemic status of secondary and tertiary health services (sufficient number of physicians and nurses, beds, intensive care beds, medical device or equipment availability)
- Status of emergency health services in terms of manpower, vehicles and equipment
- The status of the health service provision in terms of manpower, vehicle and equipment in places where people live collectively (prison, military barracks, nursing home, etc.)
- Status of workplace health services in terms of manpower, vehicle and equipment
- Personal protective equipment (PPE) availability
- Preparedness of health services at all levels for any outbreak (emergency action plan, presence of hospital disaster plan)
- Readiness of the health workforce (education, awareness)
- The nature of coordination and cooperation between all private and public health institutions
- Health Information Resources and Effective Communication
- Adequacy and availability of reliable information sources
- Health literacy level of the population
- Effective risk communication by the government
- Intersectoral Cooperation
- The nature of cooperation between non-governmental organizations, local administrations, private sector, universities, professional associations, media and central authorities

7.2 Intervention Opportunities/Capacity

- Health Services
- Coverage of diagnostic possibilities (screening in all suspicious and contacted cases and collective living places)
- Coverage of treatment options (Hospitalization opportunity for all COVID positive cases, drug supplement)

- Sufficient physical infrastructure capacity (hospital, intensive care bed, ventilator) –
- Presence of pandemic hospital practices
- The sufficient quality and quantity of health workforce involved in the battle against the outbreak
- Availability of up-to-date algorithms for case/contact management during outbreak in healthcare at all levels
- Providing qualified and sufficient PPE for health workforce
- Continuity of PPE training for newly employed staff
- Recording and monitoring the effects of healthcare workers
- Adequacy of monitoring and quarantine facilities
- Contact finding (searching for sources and contacts through all diagnosed cases) isolation and monitoring capacity (team, equipment)
- Existence of an effective surveillance system and support with information tools, compliance with WHO
- Ensuring completeness and accuracy in COVID diagnosis, treatment and death records
- Creating basic epidemiological information on the outbreak, preparing technical reports and publishing medical articles
- Sharing data in openness that allows secondary analysis
- Creating out-of-hospital isolation facilities (hotel, dormitory, building field tent)
- Proper integration of family physician facility, workplace and emergency health services via 2nd and 3rd level institutions
- Integration of health service provision in collective living areas (prison, nursing home, etc.) to outbreak management

7.2.1 Individual Precautions Regarding Disease Control

- Promotion of personal hygiene (especially hand washing and respiratory hygiene), availability of hand washing facilities in all settings
- Encouraging the use of masks, providing in adequate amounts and controlling compliance to wearing masks
- Promoting physical isolation and controlling compliance
- Promoting homestay
- Quarantine and isolation procedures

7.2.2 Social Precautions Regarding Disease Control

- Controls imposed on entering/exiting the country/cities, travel restrictions, closing of airports, quarantine application when entering the country
- Closing down workplaces and schools
- Declaring a curfew
- Banning of traffic
- Restrictions on public transport
- Restrictions on bazaar markets
- Banning of collective events
- Restriction/prohibition of public spaces/squares
- Governance
- Establishment and effective operation of the Scientific Committee
- Establishment and effective operation of pandemic provincial boards
- Effective risk communication
- Increasing access to reliable information sources

7.2.3 Bottom Phase

- Population and geographical features
- The density of risk groups (population aged 60 and over, those with chronic diseases, those who live collectively in institutions (prisons, military barracks, nursing homes), immuno-compromised persons and the number and susceptibiliity of immigrants), presence of groups in which exposure is high when by mitigating the measures and consequences will be severe
- Education, income and social security distribution of the province, existence of regions where inequalities are concentrated
- The city's capability to attract/discharge immigration (potential to receive visitors from larger cities)
- Features of working and economic life (Heavy industry, informal working conditions, child labor, seasonal work, high number of touristical businesses, etc.)
- Business of travelling (airports, airport with international flights, road mobility)
- Seasonal changes and the existence of special events (religious holidays, visiting period of immigrants, weddings, celebrations, etc.) (the effect of the disease on control measures as well as transmission routes)

7.2.4 Morbidity and Mortality Criteria

- Status of the general health indicators of the province (maternal and infant deaths, vaccination rates, etc.)
- The prevalence of the groups susceptible to coronavirus (such as DM, CHD, COPD, HT)
- Basic epidemiological information regarding the mitigation of the measures against outbreak and the availability of this information (distribution by age, location, specific groups, detailed data on test practices, contacts, treatment, isolation and quarantine processes)
- Existence of a region with a cluster of cases
- Mortality criteria (distribution of deaths by age and gender, rates specific to disease groups/risk factors, case fatality rate)
- Completeness, accuracy and transparency of all health records, especially the death registration system
- Existence of a region with a cluster of cases
- Mortality criteria (distribution of deaths by age and gender, rates specific to disease groups/risk factors, case fatality rate)
- Completeness, accuracy and transparency of all health records, especially the death registration system
- Health Services
- Extent of unmet services during the outbreak (elective operations, outpatient services, follow-ups, continuous treatments)
- The capacity to meet the service burden that will be increases after returning to routine services (the sufficient number of physicians, nurses, etc. health staff per population)
- Personal protective equipment (PPE) availability
- Health Information Sources and Effective Communication
- Adequacy and availability of reliable information sources
- Health literacy level of the population
- Effective risk communication by the government,
- Intersectoral Cooperation
- The nature of cooperation between non-governmental organizations, local administrations, private sector, universities, professional associations, media and central authorities

- Health Services
- Increasing COVID-19 awareness among people in risk groups by healthcare personnel
- Improving risk groups' access to services (COVID-19 testing and treatment)

7.2.5 Planning shifting to routine health services at all levels including primary health care

- Organizing the service provision of the groups who could not receive service during the outbreak in all steps, preventing crowding in hospitals (Telemedicine applications, examination intervals and timing that will not create congestion in the MHRS system)
- Increasing the coverage of COVID PCR tests (providing widespread test opportunities in collective living places, including asymptomatic cases)
- Increasing the rapid serological test capacity and ensuring its accessibility
- Development of monitoring systems and applications sensitive to personal rights
- Updating algorithms for case/contact management in outbreak in all levels of healthcare in line with scientific evidence
- Providing and maintaining adequate and qualified PPE for health workforce
- Continuity of PPE training for newly employed staff (new graduates, etc.)
- Planning the follow-up and control of the infected healthcare workers, existence of regulations for their personal rights
- Review of monitoring and quarantine facilities for a possible new epidemic
- Finding sufficient contacts (searching for the sources and contacts of the diagnosed people) isolation and monitoring capacity (team, equipment)
- The existence of an effective surveillance system and its support with information tools, its parallelism with WHO
- Ensuring completeness and accuracy in COVID diagnosis, treatment and death records
- Creating basic epidemiological information on the epidemic, preparing technical reports and publishing medical articles
- Sharing data in openness that allows secondary analysis
- Treatment opportunities (Hospitalization opportunity for all COVID positive cases)

7.2.6 Individual Precautions Regarding Disease Control

- Promotion of personal hygiene (especially hand washing and respiratory hygiene), availability of hand washing facilities in all environments
- Encouraging the use of masks, providing in adequate amounts and controlling compliance
- Promoting physical isolation and controlling compliance
- Promoting homestay

7.2.7 Social Precautions Regarding Disease Control

- Allowing entrances and exits to the country/city, gradual opening of airports to countries, abolishing the quarantine application after entrance
- Gradual opening of workplaces (certain days of the week, certain group workplaces)
- Maintaining physical distance at workplaces, defining rules and new practices (flexible working, rotating work, space arrangements)
- Gradual opening of schools (certain days, certain classes), determination of principles regarding the conduct of exams
- Availability of distance education/management facilities
- Gradual relaxation of the curfew (certain days, certain hours, certain groups, etc.)
- Defining the rules and new practices regarding public transportation
- Defining rules and new practices regarding bazaars and markets (crowding prevention and physical distance principles)
- Presence of new regulations regarding public areas and public transportation
- Existence of new travel regulations

7.2.8 Governance

- Efficient operation of the scientific board
- Effective work of pandemic provincial boards
- Effective risk communication
- Providing access to reliable information sources [17]

The outbreak process we are experiencing has shown that pre-epidemic socio-demographic characteristics, social infrastructure, health system capability and democracy culture, as well as combating strategies, make the struggle stronger or weaker [17]. These features function as a parameter in the risk evaluation guidelines of WHO and ECDC [37, 38]. The size of the outbreak and the change in the number of cases is shaped according to the characteristics of the agent and the route of transmission, as well as the characteristics of the society exposed to the agent and the adequacy of combatting opportunities, varying with the temporal characteristics (season, religious holidays, tourism) and geographical regions (urban–rural, metropolitan). In the battle against the virus, the status of resources at the country/local level (infrastructure, manpower, research and development etc.), preparedness, mobilizing capabilities, cooperation-coordination and participatory decision-making mechanisms in the organizational culture have gained importance [17]. In the battle against the Covid-19 virus, which has emerged with a new agent with many unknown findings, there is a need for those approaches that examine the risks with a global, national and local perspective on the basis of science and implement protective and preventive interventions in this direction.

For those countries such as Turkey having many cities with different geographical and climatic structure, populational characteristics and socio-economic conditions, there is an urgent need to be met in the risk evaluation and intervention at the provincial level. Even the regions where the risk will differ within the same province can be examined in this context. The provinces are authorized for additional measures to be taken by provincial pandemic boards, taking into account their own special circumstances [17]. In risk evaluation to be carried out at the provincial level, differences in age, socioeconomic and cultural characteristics, disadvantaged groups, collective living institutions, seasonal risks in the province should be addressed seperately, and the framework of the intervention should be transformed into a gradual mitigation by examining these risks.

Equally important, or perhaps more important thing is whether information about the outbreak is accessible. "Experts" cannot be expected to make an accurate risk evaluation without basic data and essential information. Information is one of the most important pillars of decision-making processes of both individuals and social structures. It plays an important role in perceiving a risk and developing an attitude and behavior towards a subject. Accurate and shared information also contributes to the creation of a trustful atmosphere in the society. Decision processes based on scientific data and evidence are more successful in achieving desired results on a subject. Evidence-based decision making focuses on obtaining the best (optimum) result on a subject [39].

Another important issue in outbreak management is associated with ensuring community engagement [40, 41]. International health guidelines emphasize the importance of community engagement. Combining views and insights from different segments of society is of paramount importance in enhancing the well-being. That's why healthcare professionals work with the community to plan, research, deliver and evaluate healthcare services. In the coronavirus pandemic, community engagement has been crucial in many collective responses, from compliance with the stay-at-home call to steps that countries need to take to alleviate restrictions, and help people who need support in the community through volunteering services [38]. The community wants to participate in the process [42]. This was evident during the pandemic process. Therefore, effective mechanisms should be established to include all segments of the society in outbreak management processes. Optimal results in an outbreak, a situation in which cases and deaths are minimized, fundamental rights and freedoms are protected, economic development and social life can be sustained, can only be achieved with an approach that provides transparency, evidence-based decisions, effective risk communication and community engagement [17].

Author details

Vasfiye Bayram Değer
Faculty of Health Sciences, Mardin Artuklu University, Mardin, Turkey

*Address all correspondence to: vasfiyedeg@gmail.com

IntechOpen

© 2021 The Author(s). Licensee IntechOpen. This chapter is distributed under the terms of the Creative Commons Attribution License (http://creativecommons.org/licenses/by/3.0), which permits unrestricted use, distribution, and reproduction in any medium, provided the original work is properly cited.

References

[1] Kılıç O. "Tarihte Küresel Salgın Hastalıklar ve Toplum Hayatına Etkileri", Küresel Salgının Anotomisi: İnsan ve Toplumun Geleceği, Ed.: M. Şeker, A. Özer, C.Korkut. 2020.

[2] Dinçol MA. "Ashella Rituali (CTH 394) ve Hititlerde Salgın Hastalıklara Karşı Yapılan Majik İşlemlere Toplu Bir Bakış". Türk Tarih Kurumu Belleten, XLIV. 1985; 193: 40.

[3] Ataç A, Uçar M. "Önemli Bulaşıcı Hastalıklar ve Yaşam Sürelerine Etkileri", Bilim Tarihi Araştırmaları: Salgın Hastalıklar Tarihi. 2006; 2: 33-42.

[4] Turan A, Çelikyay Hamza H. "Türkiye'de Kovid-19 ile Mücadele: Politikalar ve Aktörler", Uluslararası Yönetim Akademisi Dergisi. 2020; 3(1): 1-25.

[5] Tunç A, Atıcı FZ. Dünyada ve Türkiye'de Pandemilerle Mücadele: Risk ve Kriz Yönetimi Bağlamında Bir Değerlendirme. Troyacademy. 2020; 5 (2): 329-362.

[6] Diamond J. Tüfek, Mikrop ve Çelik, Çev.: Ü. İnce, İstanbul: Pegasus Yayınları. 2018.

[7] Türkiye Bilimler Akademisi (TÜBA). COVİD-19 Pandemi Değerlendirme Raporu, Türkiye Bilimler Akademisi Yayınları, 2020; 34: 159.

[8] Hays JN. Epidemics and Pandemics: Their Impacts on Human History, California: ABC-CLIO. 2005.

[9] Thucydides. Peloponnessos Savaşları, Çev.: F. Akderin, Belge Yayınları.2019.

[10] Özdemir H. Salgın Hastalıklardan Ölümler: 1914-1918, Türk Tarih Kurumu. 2005.

[11] Yolun M. "İspanyol Gribinin Dünya ve Osmanlı Devleti Üzerindeki Etkileri", Yüksek Lisans Tezi, Adıyaman Üniversitesi Sosyal Bilimler Enstitüsü, Adıyaman. 2012.

[12] TBD. TBD Kamu-BİB, 2006. "Bilişim Teknolojilerinde Risk Yönetimi", 2. Çalışma Grubu, Kamu Bilişim Platformu VIII, 66s. 2006.

[13] Cener P. "Kriz Yönetimi", http://danismend.com/kategori/altkategori/krizyonetimi- 1/, 2007. (Access Date: 22.08.2020).

[14] Köse H. "Yeni Risk Tanımlamaları Bağlamında Küresel Medya", Selçuk İletişim. 2007; 5(1): 42-51.

[15] Tunç A, Ağır O, Belli A, Özdemir FN. "Yönetimde Yeni Bir Yaklaşım Olarak Kriz Yönetimine Teorik Bir Bakış", VII. Uluslararası Sempozyum İdealden Gerçeğe Toplum, Siyaset ve Ekonomi, Malatya. 2018; 82-89.

[16] Özer MA. 21. Yüzyılda Yönetim ve Yöneticiler, Ankara: Nobel Basım Yayın. 2011.

[17] İnandı T, Sakarya S, Ünal B, Ergin I. "COVID-19 Salgını Özelinde Karar Vericiler için Risk Değerlendirme Yaklaşımı", Sağlık ve Toplum Dergisi (Özel Sayı). 2020; 27-38.

[18] Cadoğlu K. Risk Yönetimi ve TSK'daki Uygulamalar, İstanbul: Harp Akademileri Yayınları.2000.

[19] Emhan A. "Risk Yönetim Süreci ve Risk Yönetmekte Kullanılan Teknikler", Atatürk Üniversitesi İktisadi ve İdari bilimler Dergisi. 2009; 23(3): 209-220.

[20] Sezgin F. "Kriz Yönetimi", Gazi Üniversitesi Sosyal Bilimler Dergisi. 2003; 4(8): 181-195.

[21] Porzio G, Cortellini A, Bruera E, Verna L, Ravoni G, Peris F et al. Home Care for Cancer Patients During

COVID-19 Pandemic: The Double Triage Protocol. 9-11 J Pain Symptom Manage. 2020 Jul; 60(1): e5-e7. doi: 10.1016/j.jpainsymman.2020.03.021.

[22] İşsever H, İşsever T, Öztan G. Epidemiology of COVID-19. Sağlık Bilimlerinde İleri Araştırmalar Dergisi. 2020; 3(1): 2-13. DOI: 10.26650/JARHS2020-S1-0001.

[23] Zheng S, Fan J, Yu F, Feng B, Lou B, Zou Q, et al. Viral load dynamics and disease severity in patients infected with SARS-CoV-2 in Zhejiang province, China, January-March 2020. BMJ; 369. doi: 10.1136/bmj.m1443.

[24] Şengül E, Ünal E. COVID-19 Salgınında Halk Sağlığı Yönetimi. Med Res Rep. 2020; 3(Supp 1): 162-171.

[25] WHO.Clinical management of severe acute respiratory infection (SARI) when COVID-19 disease is suspected: interim guidance, 2020. World Health Organization, 2020.

[26] Adhikari SP, Meng S, Wu Y-J, Mao Y-P, Ye R-X, Wang Q-Z, et al. Epidemiology, causes, clinical manifestation and diagnosis, prevention and control of coronavirus disease (COVID-19) during the early outbreak period: a scoping review. Infectious Diseases Of Poverty. 2020; 9(1): 1-12.

[27] WHO. Novel Coronavirus (2019-nCoV) Situation Report–11. (2020). https://www.who.int/docs/default-source/coronaviruse/situation-reports/20200131-sitrep-11-ncov.pdf?sfvrsn=de7c0f7_4. Access date: 21 Jan 2020.

[28] Ceylan Z. Estimation of COVID-19 prevalence in Italy, Spain, and France. Sci Total Environ.2020; 729: 138817. doi:10.1016/j.scitotenv.2020.138817

[29] Mavragani A. Tracking COVID-19 in Europe: Infodemiology Approach. JMIR Public Health Surveill. 2020; 6(2): e18941. Published 2020 Apr 20. doi:10.2196/18941

[30] Bashir MF, Faroog TM, BEN JİAN Ma, Komal B et al. Correlation between environmental pollution indicators and COVID-19 pandemic: A brief study in Californian context. Enviromental Research. 2020; 728: 138.835. https://doi.org/10.1016/j.envres.2020.109652.

[31] Worldometer. Covid-19 Coronavirus Pandemic. https://www.worldometers.info/coronavirus/. (Acces Date: 27 Dec 2020).

[32] T.C. Sağlık Bakanlığı COVİD-19 Rehberi. https://covid19bilgi.saglik.gov.tr/tr/covid- 19-rehberi.html / (Erişim Tarihi: 27.06.2020).

[33] Samancı VM. Birinci Basamak Sağlık Hizmetleri ve Pandemi Süreci. Konuralp Tıp Dergisi. 2020; 12(S1): 391-393.

[34] Sağlık Bakanlığı Bilim Kurulu Çalışma Kılavuzu. Temaslı Takibi, Salgın Yönetimi, Evde Hasta İzlemi Ve Filyasyon, Ankara. 01. 06. 2020

[35] Wikipedia, "Basic reproduction number-Wikipedia." https://en.wikipedia.org/wiki/Basic_reproduction_number (Acces Date: 27.05.2020).

[36] N.C.I. Centers for Disease Control and Prevention, "Implementation of Mitigation Strategies for Communities with Local COVID-19 Transmission." https://www.cdc.gov/coronavirus/2019-ncov/downloads/community-mitigation-strategy.pdf. (Acces Date: 27.05. 2020).

[37] WHO. World Health Organization, Rapid Risk Assessment of Acute Public Health Events. 2012.

[38] ECDC. European Centre for Disease Prevention and Control. Technical Document:Operational

guidance on rapid risk assessment methodology. 2011.

[39] Wikipedia. (2020). “Knowledge-based decision making - Wikipedia.” https://en.wikipedia.org/wiki/Knowledge-based_decision_making. (Acces Date: 27.05.2020).

[40] UNAIDS. (2020). UNAIDS “Rights in the time of COVID-19 — Lessons from HIV for an effective, community-led response | UNAIDS.” https://www.unaids.org/en/resources/documents/2020/human-rights-and-covid-19. (Acces Date: 27. 05. 2020).

[41] World Health Organization. “WHO | Global Strategy for Women’s, Children’s and Adolescent’s Health & Every Woman Every Child Initiative.” https://www.who.int/life- course/partners/global-strategy/en/ (Acces Date: 27.05.2020).

[42] Villadiego L. “Spaniards find beauty in helping each other amid COVID-19 crisis | Europe | Al Jazeera.” https://www.aljazeera.com/indepth/features/spaniards-find-beauty- helping-covid-19-crisis-200319105933362.html (Acces Date: 27.05.2020).

Chapter 10

Epidemiology of Obesity in Children and Adolescents

Giulio Nittari, Stefania Scuri, Getu Gamo Sagaro, Fabio Petrelli and Iolanda Grappasonni

Abstract

The childhood overweight and obesity epidemic has become a global emergency in public health and a crucial challenge of the twenty-first century. Nowadays, childhood and adolescent obesity represent a significant public health problem both in developing and developed countries. Globally, above 340 million children and adolescents aged 5–19 years were overweight or obese in 2016. Childhood obesity is a critical burden because it can be associated with a higher possibility of obesity, premature death, and disability in adults, as well as early markers of cardiovascular disease. In Europe, childhood obesity remains a significant health challenge and is distributed disparately across and between countries and population groups. In 2019, over 398,000 children aged 6–9 years were severely obese in Europe. Particularly, Southern European countries such as Greece, Italy, Malta, San Marino, and Spain had one in five children obese in 2018. In Europe, different initiatives and actions have been launched in recent years to fight childhood obesity. However, the progress on combating obesity in children has been slow and inconsistent across the region. In this chapter, we have discussed the prevalence of obesity in children and existing policies to combat childhood obesity in the World Health Organization (WHO) European Region.

Keywords: obesity, overweight, childhood, adolescents, prevalence, epidemiology, policies, prevention

1. Introduction

Obesity in children is the most serious public health problem globally [1], as children are more likely to become obese adults in their future lives. Currently, childhood obesity represents a significant public health challenge in both developed and developing countries by increasing the burden of noncommunicable diseases (NCDs) [2]. Recent estimates suggest that over 38 million children younger than 5 years of age were overweight or obese in 2019 [3]. Over 340 million children and adolescents aged 5–19 years were overweight or obese in 2016 [3]. The prevention of diabetes mellitus and obesity in adults and children was one of the goals set by the World Health Assembly in 2013 [4]. The rapid increase worldwide in obesity is also analyzed in association with the economic causes because some differences were observed between high- and low-income settings. In high-income settings, the higher prevalence of obesity is observed in disadvantaged and marginalized communities. In contrast, in low- and middle-income settings, the prevalence of obesity is higher in groups with higher socioeconomic status. This trend can be explained by socioeconomic inequalities, because in the high-income countries, commonly, the socioeconomic disparities improve the consumption by the poor people of inexpensive, energy-dense foods and beverages.

Furthermore, the increment of obesity prevalence by 23–33% was recorded for children in low-education, low-income, and higher-unemployment households. The family with low-income demonstrates a lower awareness that their children are overweight and then face a host of barriers to improving the diet, the activity behaviors, and the general health status [5]. Many economic consequences for public health strategies are related to the epidemic trend of childhood obesity.

The problem of childhood obesity has become a global public health concern, and the fight for its prevention is a commitment that involves all institutions. The prevention of obesity requires the implementation of surveys to monitor its evolution over time, the knowledge of its determinants, and the research and implementation of interventions, necessarily in a multisectoral and multidisciplinary context, as well as a continuous evaluation process. These actions are necessary for the implementation of evidence-based interventions, which must be supported by appropriate nutritional policies. Overweight and obesity at a young age are associated with various health or economic consequences, therefore it is important to analyze the causes and risk factors and identify the best prevention and treatment strategies. On the prevention of childhood obesity, the promotion of teamwork and the dissemination of information related to childhood obesity is one of the vital strategies to fight against childhood and adolescent obesity. Therefore, teamwork in health care is a crucial strategy for promoting public health and preventing childhood chronic diseases such as childhood obesity.

In Europe, childhood obesity remains a significant health challenge and is distributed disparately across and between countries and population groups [6]. Approximately, 398, 000 children aged 6–9 years were severely obese in Europe in 2019 [7]. Obesity in children is associated with immediate adverse consequences such as psychological problems [8] and lower educational attainment [9]. Also, it is associated with negative health effects later in life or adulthood, such as type 2 diabetes mellitus, hypertension, obstructive sleep apnea, dyslipidemia, and other noncommunicable diseases [10]. Childhood obesity is the outcome of an interaction between a complex series of factors related to environmental, genetic, and ecological effects [10]. Due to the speedily increasing prevalence of childhood obesity in Europe, various initiatives and actions have been launched in recent years in response to this alarming trend. As a result, the WHO European Childhood Obesity Surveillance Initiative has measured the trends in childhood obesity for over a decade [11]. It provides data to inform policy and practice to respond to the problem of childhood obesity [11, 12]. Also, the EU developed an action plan to tackle childhood obesity (EU Action Plan on Childhood Obesity 2014–2020) on February 24, 2014 [13]. However, the progress on combating obesity in children has been slow and inconsistent across the region. For instance, the latest data have shown that southern European countries such as Greece, Italy, Malta, Cyprus, San Marino, and Spain have the highest rate of childhood obesity (nearly one in five children are obese) [14]. On the other hand, Denmark, France, Ireland, and Norway are among countries with the lowest rates of obesity in children in either sex [14]. Hence, childhood obesity is still a so-called time bomb [15] for future demands for health services and could jeopardize the progress toward achieving the Sustainable Development Goals (SDGs) [16].

The present chapter is aimed at (1) illustrating the prevalence of obesity in children and adolescents aged 5—19 years by the WHO European Region and (2) analyzing the effectiveness of the prevention strategies adopted in EU countries to combat childhood obesity from a social and legal point of view and pointing out the best strategies to reduce the prevalence of obesity in children and adolescents.

2. Epidemiology

2.1 Prevalence

Data on the prevalence of obesity in children and adolescents aged 5—19 years in the WHO European Region were taken from the Global Health Observatory (GHO) data [17]. By geographic area, the highest crude prevalence of childhood obesity was observed in Mediterranean countries in 2016, ranging from 7.6% to 13.8% for either sex. In particular, Greece, Malta, Italy, Cyprus, Andorra, Turkey, and Israel among the Mediterranean countries had the highest prevalence of childhood and adolescent obesity in 2016 (**Table 1**). In 1980, Oriental European countries had a prevalence of less than 2%, ranging from 0.3 to 1.9%. However, in 2016, it changed completely, and the prevalence was more than 4%, ranging from 4.2 to 11.1% (**Table 1**). The prevalence in all northern European countries, except Iceland, increased by over 100% between 1980 and 2016, but in Iceland, it increased by 94% in the same period (5.1% in 1980 and 9.9% in 2016). In 2016, among the Western European countries, the United Kingdom (UK) and Germany had the highest childhood obesity. In contrast, Armenia, Azerbaijan, and the Republic of Moldova among Eastern European countries with relatively low prevalence levels (**Table 1**). The prevalence distribution in Oriental Europe countries showed relatively small when compared to the other areas in Europe in 2016. However, EU member states (Bulgaria, Czechia, Hungary, Lithuania, Poland, Slovakia) among Oriental countries had higher prevalence levels (**Table 1**).

2.2 Trends

Obesity in children aged 5–19 years in almost all European regions have increased rapidly from 1980 to 2016. Mainly EU member states have shown increasing trends in the prevalence of obesity in children and adolescents during the study period. Notably, Greece and Croatia have shown secular trends in the prevalence of childhood obesity among EU countries in the Mediterranean Region (**Figure 1**). Besides, the prevalence in the United Kingdom tripled for either sex from 1980 to 2016, ranging from 3.4 to 10.2%, respectively (**Table 1**). Similarly, in France and Spain, the prevalence almost tripled from 1980 to 2016: for example, in France, it ranged from 3% in 1980 to 8.1% in 2016 and in Spain, passing from 3.8% in 1980 to 10.8% in 2016 (**Table 1**). In Slovakia, the prevalence of obesity in children has increased from 0.6% in 1980 to 8.1% in 2016 (**Table 1**). On the other hand, in Cyprus, Lithuania, Portugal, and the Netherlands, the prevalence has increased more than five times over 36 years in each country (**Table 1**). In contrast, in Italy, Malta, and Belgium, the magnitude of childhood obesity has doubled from 1980 to 2016. As shown in **Table 1**, in Poland, the prevalence has increased from 1% in 1980 to 9.1% in 2016, while in Bulgaria, it grew by more than eight times in the same

	1980			1990			2000			2010			2016		
	M (%)	F (%)	T (%)	M (%)	F (%)	T (%)	M (%)	F (%)	T (%)	M (%)	F (%)	T (%)	M (%)	F (%)	T (%)
Mediterranean Region															
Turkey	0.7	0.8	0.7	2.3	2.5	2.4	5.2	5.3	5.2	9.3	8.7	9	12.1	10.9	11.5
Cyprus	3.7	1.8	2.7	8.5	4.2	6.4	11.9	6.1	9.1	14.1	7.6	10.9	15.5	8.7	12.2
Israel	7.5	5.9	6.7	9.8	7	8.4	11.8	8.1	10	13.4	9	11.3	14.2	9.5	11.9
Andorra	8.8	7	7.9	11.9	8.6	10.3	13.4	9.3	11.4	14.5	10	12.3	15	10.4	12.8
Malta	8.6	7.2	7.9	11.2	8.2	9.8	13.2	9.4	11.4	14.9	10.5	12.7	15.7	11.1	13.4
Portugal	2	1.7	1.9	4.4	3.5	3.9	7.9	6.4	7.2	10.4	9.2	9.8	10.7	10.2	10.4
Spain	4.7	2.8	3.8	7	3.8	5.4	9.3	5.1	7.3	11.8	7.2	9.5	13.1	8.4	10.8
Albania	0.4	0.2	0.3	1	0.6	0.8	2.6	1.5	2.1	6.1	3.6	4.9	9.5	5.5	7.6
Croatia	1.3	0.7	1	3.1	1.7	2.4	5.9	3.2	4.6	10.3	5.7	8.1	13.8	7.9	10.9
France	3.2	2.9	3	4.5	3.7	4.1	6.2	5	5.6	7.9	6.3	7.1	8.9	7.2	8.1
Greece	5.8	3.6	4.7	8.5	4.9	6.7	11.2	6.6	9	14.8	9.1	12	16.8	10.7	13.8
Italy	6.2	4.2	5.2	8.2	5.1	6.7	12.2	7.2	9.3	13.3	9.3	11.4	14.5	10.4	12.5
Montenegro	0.4	0.2	0.3	1.3	0.7	1	3.7	2	2.9	7.2	3.9	5.6	9.7	5.3	7.6
Northern Region															
Iceland	5.8	4.4	5.1	8.2	5.5	6.9	10.2	6.3	8.1	11.5	6.7	9.1	12.5	7.2	9.9
Ireland	1.4	1.5	1.5	3	3.1	3.1	5.3	5.6	5.4	8.5	8	8.3	10.4	9.1	9.8
Denmark	3.7	3.3	3.5	6	4.5	5.3	8.1	5.2	6.7	8.8	4.9	6.9	9.4	4.9	7.2
Estonia	1.7	1.7	1.7	2.6	2.3	2.5	3.6	2.8	3.2	5.6	3.7	4.7	7.8	4.7	6.3
Finland	3.4	1.5	2.5	6.7	3	4.9	9.3	4.2	6.8	11.1	4.9	8.1	12.4	5.6	9.1

	1980			1990			2000			2010			2016		
	M (%)	F (%)	T (%)	M (%)	F (%)	T (%)	M (%)	F (%)	T (%)	M (%)	F (%)	T (%)	M (%)	F (%)	T (%)
Netherlands	1.4	1.2	1.3	2.5	2	2.3	4.5	3.4	3.9	6.9	4.8	5.9	8.4	5.6	7
Norway	2.7	2.5	2.6	4.7	3.9	4.3	7.2	5.6	6.4	9.1	6.8	8	10.4	7.7	9.1
Sweden	3.3	2.5	2.9	4.7	2.9	3.9	6.5	3.6	5	7.4	4	5.7	8.6	4.7	6.7
Oriental Region															
Hungary	2	1.4	1.7	3.5	2.3	2.9	5.8	3.7	4.8	9.9	6.2	8.1	13.7	8.4	11.1
Kazakhstan	1.5	0.8	1.2	2.4	1.4	1.9	3.7	2.1	2.9	5.6	3.4	4.6	8.1	4.9	6.5
Lithuania	1.3	1.1	1.2	2.7	2.1	2.4	4.3	2.8	3.6	6.3	3.7	5	8.7	4.8	6.8
Armenia	1.3	1.2	1.3	2.2	1.9	2	2.8	2.3	2.6	3.8	3.2	3.5	5.3	4.2	4.8
Azerbaijan	0.9	0.7	0.8	1.5	1.2	1.3	2.2	1.8	2	3.5	2.9	3.2	5.3	4.4	4.9
Bosnia and Herzegovina	0.3	0.2	0.3	1	0.6	0.8	2.2	1.3	1.8	4.5	2.9	3.7	6.5	4.3	5.4
Bulgaria	1.6	1	1.3	3.4	2	2.7	5.9	3.5	4.7	10.1	5.8	8	13.6	7.8	10.8
Czech Republic	2.3	1.5	1.9	3.7	2.2	3	5.8	3.1	4.5	9.1	4.8	7	12.6	6.6	9.7
Poland	1.4	0.6	1	2.9	1.3	2.1	4.9	2.1	3.6	8.8	3.6	6.3	12.7	5.3	9.1
Republic of Macedonia	1.3	0.7	1	2.8	1.4	2.1	5.3	2.7	4	8.7	4.5	6.7	11.9	6.4	9.3
Republic of Moldova	0.4	0.3	0.4	1.1	0.8	1	2	1.4	1.7	3.2	2.1	2.7	5.1	3.3	4.2
Romania	0.8	0.4	0.6	1.7	1	1.4	3.6	1.9	2.8	7.1	3.7	5.4	10.7	5.4	8.1
Russian Federation	1.7	1.4	1.5	3.1	2.2	2.6	4.1	2.4	3.2	6.6	3.3	5	9.5	4.4	7.1

	1980			1990			2000			2010			2016		
	M (%)	F (%)	T (%)	M (%)	F (%)	T (%)	M (%)	F (%)	T (%)	M (%)	F (%)	T (%)	M (%)	F (%)	T (%)
Serbia	1	0.5	0.8	2.5	1.2	1.9	5.1	2.5	3.8	9.2	4.9	7.1	12.4	7	9.8
Slovakia	0.8	0.4	0.6	1.8	1	1.4	3.5	1.9	2.7	6.8	3.7	5.3	10.4	5.7	8.1
Occidental Region															
Switzerland	1.1	0.9	1	3.1	2.1	2.6	5	3.1	4.1	6	3.8	5	6.9	4.6	5.8
United Kingdom	3	3.8	3.4	5.2	6	5.6	8.3	8.6	8.5	10.3	9.6	9.9	10.9	9.4	10.2
Luxembourg	3.6	2.7	3.2	5.7	3.8	4.8	7.8	4.9	6.4	9.5	5.7	7.6	10.4	6.2	8.3
Belgium	4.5	4.6	4.6	6.3	5.2	5.8	7.5	5.6	6.6	7.8	5.5	6.7	8.2	5.8	7
Austria	3.5	1.8	2.6	5.6	2.6	4.1	7.9	3.6	5.8	9.8	4.8	7.4	11.2	6	8.6
Germany	3.8	2.7	3.3	5.9	3.7	4.9	8	4.8	6.4	9.7	5.8	7.8	11	6.8	8.9

Data source: Global Health Observatory (GHO) data [17]; M, male; F, female; and T, total.

Table 1.
Prevalence (%) of obesity in children aged 5–19 years by the WHO European region from 1980 to 2016.

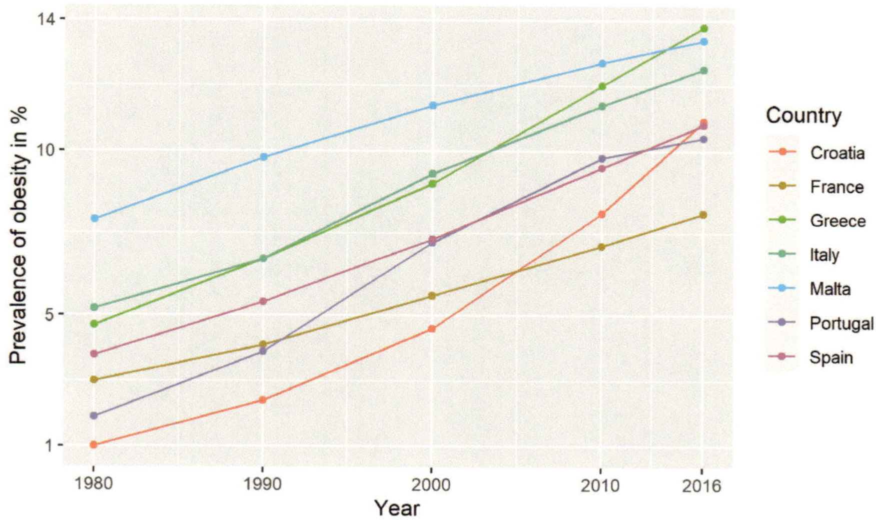

Figure 1.
Trends in the prevalence of obesity in children and adolescents aged between 5 and 19 years in the Mediterranean region EU countries from 1980 to 2016.

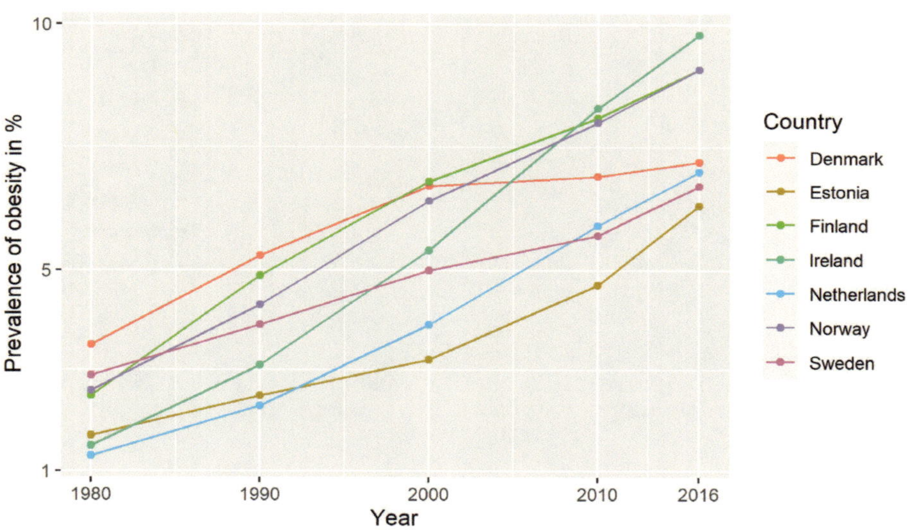

Figure 2.
Trends in the prevalence of obesity in children and adolescents aged between 5 and 19 years in the northern EU countries from 1980 to 2016.

period (1.3% in 1980 and 10.8% in 2016). In Ireland, the prevalence of obesity in children and adolescents has steadily increased over 36 years (1.5% in 1980 and 9.8% in 2016) (**Figure 2**). Mainly the prevalence level increased from 1.5 and 1.4%, respectively, for girls and boys in 1980 to 9.1 and 10.4% for girls and boys in 2016 (**Table 1**). Furthermore, the Oriental EU member states except for Lithuania all have shown consistently increased trends in the prevalence over 16 years (from 2000 to 2016) (**Figure 3**). Trends in the prevalence of obesity in children and adolescents aged 5–19 years have been presented in EU countries by geographic areas (**Figures 1–4**).

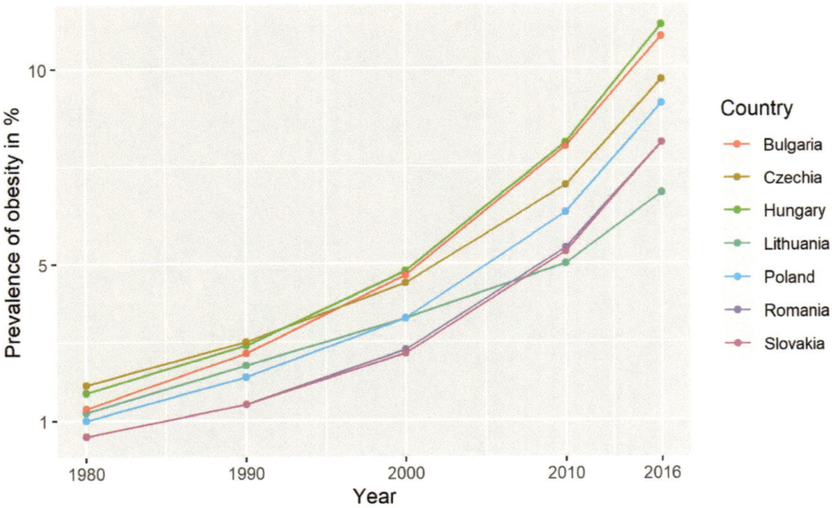

Figure 3.
Trends in the prevalence of obesity in children and adolescents aged between 5 and 19 years in the oriental EU countries from 1980 to 2016.

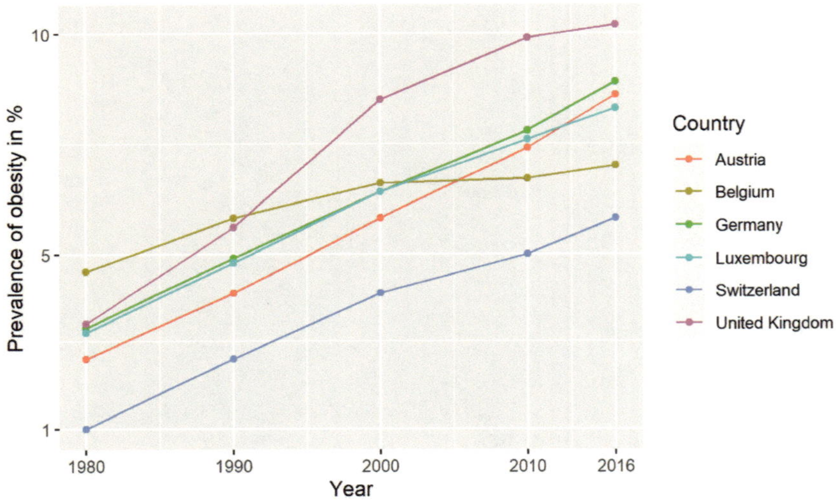

Figure 4.
Trends in the prevalence of obesity in children and adolescents aged between 5 and 19 years in the occidental EU countries from 1980 to 2016.

3. Policies

The alarming proportions reached by childhood obesity in many countries pose an urgent and serious challenge, also concerning the most serious consequences of obesity on health. Obesity can produce effects immediately on a child's health, educational performance, and quality of life, or chronic illnesses in adults, which are very likely to remain obese. The policy to tack childhood obesity is slow and inconsistent and then to review and resolve this gap, in 2014, the Commission on Ending Childhood obesity has been established. Moreover, the "Strengthening Nutrition Action of Food and Agriculture Organization of the United Nations and World Health Organization-United Nations decade of Action on Nutrition 2016-2025," describes that in the same year (2014). The Second International Conference on Nutrition (ICN2) listed obesity and overweight among the malnutrition forms. It focused the attention of 164 member States of FAO and WHO, about the need to change the choices of the food systems for better diets and a healthier planet. The unhealthy diets, maternal and child malnutrition, are considered as the current top risk factors for one-quarter of global deaths.

Furthermore, the number of people of all ages who are affected by diet-related noncommunicable diseases (NCDs) has increased. The documents produced by ICN2 make up the roadmap for the governments of the world to eradicate hunger and prevent all forms of malnutrition such as undernutrition, micronutrient deficiency, overweight, and obesity. One year later, has been adopted the 2030 Agenda for Sustainable Development ("2023 Agenda") and its Sustainable Development Goals (SDGs) at the United Nations (UN) General Assembly. In 2015, the United Nations mentioned the prevention and control of noncommunicable diseases as a top priority in the Sustainable Development Goals, and obesity listed as a risk factor for noncommunicable diseases [18]. The Global Action Plan for the Prevention and Control of Non-communicable Diseases 2013–2020 assess policy options for member states per their legislation for the selection and for undertaking actions from among the policy options about the monitoring, the disease registries, and the surveillance of NCDs.

Regarding the surveillance, the WHO indicates the surveillance of the key risk for the NCDs considering behavioral and metabolic risk factors as for example the use of alcohol, the physical inactivity, tobacco use, unhealthy diet, overweight, and obesity, raised blood pressure, raised blood glucose, and hyperlipidemia, and determinants of risk exposure such as marketing of food, tobacco, and alcohol [19]. Moreover, to accelerate the actions on nutrition, the UN General Assembly, in 2016, proposed that the period from 2016 to 2020 should be a UN Decade of Action on Nutrition (Nutrition Decade), providing a clearly defined, time-bound, and cohesive framework for all countries and stakeholders to increase nutrition investments and implement policies and programs to improve food security and nutrition, reach the six global nutrition targets 2025, and the diet-related global noncommunicable disease (NCD) targets. Modifying possible risk factors as the reduction of an unhealthy diet is one of the "best buys" for the prevention and control of noncommunicable diseases (NCDs) proposed by the World Health Organization [20].

All reports proposed by the international organization of public health proposed a no single intervention to resolve childhood obesity and overweight but analyses and interventions about the environmental context and three critical periods in the life-course. The first is the preconception and pregnancy, infancy and early childhood, and finally, older childhood and adolescence. Therefore, the prevention and the treatment of obesity require a whole-of-government approach in which the policies of all sectors are across the same target, which the health, the eradication of harmful health impacts, and thus improve population health and health equity. The Commission on Ending Childhood Obesity collected and an organic package of recommendations to address childhood obesity and achieve strategic objectives. As a result, the first object is tacking the obesogenic environment because the major negative elements are the unhealthy diet and physical activity of children. The second goal is the reduction of the risk to develop the obesity development factors able to change the biology and behavior of children before birth and through infancy. The last is the treatment and cure of children or young people with notified obesity. Consequently, the areas identified by the commission to define the preventive actions are the promotion of healthy foods intake, physical activity, the cure preconception, and pregnancy care, the early childhood diet, and physical activity, the health, nutrition, and physical activity for school-age children and finally the weight management. The first recommendation concerns the promotion of healthy food intake and the reduction of sugar-sweetened beverages by children and adolescents. Among the actions promoted are listed the development and diffusion of appropriate and context-specific nutrition guidelines for adults and children, the implementation of a tax on sugar-sweetened beverages, and the marketing of foods and nonalcoholic beverages to children. Besides, the description of the nutrient-profiles to identify unhealthy foods and beverages associated with a standardized global nutrient labeling system. The Codex Alimentarius Commission proposes a standardized system of food labeling for all packaged foods and beverages, which can support the nutrition and health education [21]. In association with the correct labeling system could be improved, also, the public education of both adults and children about nutrition literacy and the interpretation of front-of-pack. This recommendation is included in the recommendation 14 of United Nations decade of Action on Nutrition 2016–2025, concerning saturated fat, sugars, salt, and trans-fat reduction has been focused on the promotion of a healthy diet to stop the consumption and sale of highly processed foods, growing fastest in lower-middle-income countries. The actions to prevent and control NCDs include the reduction of salt intake, and the setting of target levels for the amount of salt, reformulating food products. Furthermore, the action plan has been indicated the elimination of industrial trans-fats and the reduction of sugar consumption through taxation on sugar-sweetened beverages. The availability, and consequently, the high consumption of these products, is the principal cause of health problems such as obesity and other diet related NCDs. The reduction of sedentary behaviors in children and adolescents, focusing on physical activity programs, is the second recommendation and includes the definition of advice to children, adolescents, parents, caregivers, teachers, and health professionals on healthy body size, physical activity, sleep behaviors and appropriate use of screen-based entertainment. The same recommendation promotes the improvement, during the recreational time, for all children (including the children with disabilities), of physical activity favoring adequate facilities at school or in public areas. Recent epidemiologic data show a decline from the age of school about physical activity. About 81% of adolescents have insufficient physical activity lower than 60 minutes each day. Obesity is more linked with physical activity because it creates a vicious cycle, which increases body fat levels and decreases physical activity. The recommendation about the prevention of childhood overweight and obesity regarding all guidelines promoted introduces the protection of the diet in women during pregnancy, the improvement of child nutrition status and growth, and finally, the promotion of physical activity to address sedentary lifestyle from the early stages of life. The best keys to these recommendations are breastfeeding promotion and protection because they have a crucial role in the reduction of childhood obesity risk. Indeed, the diagnosis and management of hyperglycemia and gestational hypertension, the monitoring of gestational weight gain, the correct diet, and lifestyles during pregnancy are key preventive factors against childhood overweight and obesity. To ensure healthy child development, policies should provide advice not only on healthy eating but also on appropriate sleep time, sedentary or screen time, physical activity, or active play for the age group of 2–5 years. The school is also a fundamental environment to promote the correct lifestyles, especially about the diet. Two aspects can be improved at school, the promotion of standardized meals, in accordance with guidelines, without unhealthy foods with sugar, sweetened beverages or energy-dense, nutrient-poor foods etc. but characterized by the introduction of fresh fruits, vegetables, and safe drinking water. The secondary aspect is the improvement of knowledge's on children about health education within the core curriculum of schools and practical experiences of food preparation available to children, their parents, and caregivers.

Finally, the six recommendations of the commission are the correct weight management in children and young people suffering from obesity and overweight, developing multicomponent services concerning physical activity, nutrition, and psychological support. These supports are delivered by professional and treated teams, as part of Universal health coverage. The responsibilities of these actions are divided by different structures at different levels. The first is the WHO and concerns the institutionalization of each measure across all technical areas of WHO, and regional and country offices. Furthermore, it provides the consultation and technical support for action at global, regional, and national levels, with international agencies, and the governments of each Member States. Each Member States are supported by International organizations, and define political commitment against childhood obesity, coordinate all sectors and institutions engaged for policies about nutrition, food, agriculture, sport and recreation, urban planning etc. Collect and record all data on BMI-for-age of children and define the national targets for childhood obesity. The other structures are represented by nongovernmental organizations (NGOs), the private sector, the philanthropic foundations, and academic institutions [22].

In Europe, the EU Action Plan on Childhood Obesity 2014–2020 translates the international guidelines with the purpose of demonstrating the shared of EU Member States to addressing childhood obesity; set out priority areas for action and a possible toolbox of measures for consideration and finally propose ways of collectively keeping track of progress. The EU Action Plan considers the presence of three types of stakeholders which are: the 28 EU Member States, the European Commission, and international organizations such as the WHO and finally civil society (e.g., nongovernmental organizations (NGOs), industry, research institutes, and associations). The national, regional, and local level was represented by the specific authorities. Each area defined in the EU action plan is in agreement with the areas proposed by the Global Action Plan, and to evaluate the efficacy of the intervention for each region were defined as specific indicators. Regarding the area for action 1: Support a healthy start in life the first operational objective is, for example, increase the prevalence of children that are breastfed, the indicator is the % of children breastfed and the final target the achievement of 20% in 2020 of children with adequate periods of exclusive breastfeeding according to national recommendations. The area of action 2 is about the promotion of healthier environments, especially at schools and preschools, and the main priority is the establishment of children's health as a priority at schools, and for example, the first operational objective is to "provide the healthy option and increase daily consumption of fresh fruit and vegetables, healthy food and water intake in schools (with a targeted focus on schools in underprivileged districts)." The action is the development of preschool and school meals with fruits, vegetables, and drinking milk following the existing EU guidelines. The indicators are, for example, the number of member states implementing frameworks on preschool and school meals, and the target to achieve in 2020 is 90% of the member states participating in the program. The other areas are the improvement of healthy options regarding the availability of healthy food choices to children and the target of restriction related to vending machines. Area number 4 has the goal to limit the exposure of children to advertisements for food/drinks high in fat, sugars, and salt. The improvement of family knowledge and information's on the daily food and health choices of children of action number 5. The last two areas of action are number 6 to encourage physical activity, and number 7 is related to the monitoring and evaluation of children's nutritional status and behaviors. At this moment, the assessment of the effectiveness of the Action Plan that can be analyzed is referred to in 2018, because the final assessment will be defined at the end of 2020. The initial results compare the activities improved before 2014 with the activities promoted with the EU Action Plan in each action area [23]. The results show an improvement of actions relatively the guidance around the pregnancy, the policies on vending machines, energy drinks, and reformulation of food and especially the concentration of salt.

4. Prevention strategies adopted by European states

Despite the important engagement of the European countries in reversing the progress of obesity, the incidence of overweight subjects remains alarming, particularly if considering the young population. Childhood weight gain has, in fact, a severe impact on health and psychosocial outcomes, deeply affecting individual and family's quality of life. Research shows that overweight children are more likely if compared to normal weight ones, to become obese adults and so to develop chronic conditions. The recent increment of hours dedicated to "screen time" and the associated damaging effects on eating habits, together with little safe spaces to be active in, are essential factors influencing the level of physical activity and health among young. Also, cheaper and larger-portioned fast food, as well as the massive consumption of high-sugar products, must be taken into consideration. In 2014, in EU, the 7% of yearly national health budgets were spent on diseases correlated to obesity, and investigations showed how policies addressed to children obesity control would repay on investment of 6–10%.

For these reasons, in 2007, after analyzing the report by the WHO European Childhood Obesity Surveillance Initiative (COSI), the European Commission adopted the White Paper on a Strategy for Europe on Nutrition, Overweight and Obesity-related Health issues, composed of six major goals: better-informed subjects, physical activity, and healthier options promotion, supporting low socioeconomic groups and developing evidence and monitoring systems to support the program. The High-Level Group on Nutrition and Physical Activity and the EU Platform for Action on Diet, Physical Activity, and Health are the main instruments set up for implementation of the strategy. The first one enables governments to share health and economic analysis and enhances contact between governments and the EU platform for action on a diet, physical activity, and health. It also works on some priorities such as reducing children's exposure to marketing of foods high in fat, salt and sugars, physical activity, labeling, and public procurement of food, reducing health inequalities. The EU Platform is a forum for European level organizations, including Food business and consumer organizations, scientific associations, and NGOs. The high-level group can also be asked by the commission to prepare the groundwork for relevant prevention and promotion initiatives agreed by the steering group on promotion and prevention.

In 2013 the strategy went through an external evaluation to test its efficiency: the results were positive. However, they suggested a greater commitment to promoting physical activity. Besides, an Action Plan on Childhood Obesity addressed to a Europe-wide context was redacted, to lower young overweight by 2020. One of its main goals is to support a healthy start in life, encouraging breastfeeding and promoting the adoption of a healthy lifestyle both during the early stage of life and preconception period. Developing healthier school environments is the sequel, providing wholesome meals, with the proper nutritional intake, and also allowing adequate time to consume it. Making the healthy option more available in addition, both in schools and in the working environment, would encourage good eating behavior to be part of the routine. The fourth point is about making families informed in order to empower parents in planning a correct meal plan and schedule regular active leisure activities, which is also linked to the significant focus on the promotion of the physical activity. Last, the increase in monitoring and research, would, in the end, test the nutritional quality of food, health status, and habits of children, together with the collection of systematic data.

The main actors of the plan are 28 EU Member States, the European Commission, and a variety of civil society stakeholders such as NGOs, industry and agricultural sectors, University and research institutes. Another project, the Joint Action on Nutrition and Physical Activity (JANPA), was proposed as a contribution to the EU action plan on childhood obesity 2014–2020, focusing on specific outcomes that can effectively contribute to nutritional and physical activity policies during childhood. It has the following objectives: economic evaluation of the cost of overweight and obesity in children with the aim to encourage public actions, promoting healthy nutrition and physical activity to pregnant women and families with young children, promoting healthier environments in schools and preschools, efforts at a local or at a national level regarding nutrition and physical activities, promoting healthy eating and drinking practices, and improving the information addressed to the consumer at the national level [13]. At the national level, many policies and programs have been adopted in recent years in Europe, aiming to prevent child obesity and improve its treatment and management.

4.1 Italy

Data from the Childhood Obesity Surveillance Initiative (2015–17) show that Italy is ranked first in Europe for child obesity, with 21% of children obese or overweight: taking into account this evidence, Italy has turned its attention not only to monitoring, but also to the population approach, using media, brochures, and education in schools and health-care facilities. These actions are part of the Italian Health Plan on Prevention. One of the objectives of this program is to reduce the preventable and avoidable burden of morbidity, mortality, and disability of noncommunicable diseases. Another initiative adopted in Italy is the program named "OKKIO all Salute," launched in 2007 as a part of the COSI initiative, to monitor children's weight, eating behaviors, physical activity habits, and their related risk factors among children of 6–10 years. From 2008, around 45.000 families took part in this project. Italy is also part of the international program HBSC (Health Behavior in School-aged Children), showing commitment to understanding factors influencing children's eating behaviors [24].

4.2 Malta

The increasing prevalence of overweight and obesity, especially among children, is a significant public health problem in Malta, as it has been estimated that 40% of school-aged children are overweight or obese. Different actions have been put in place to tackle this problem since the Maltese Presidency of the Council of the EU selected childhood obesity as one of its priority areas during its European Presidency in the first half of 2017. Considering the fact that children spend much time in school, particular attention was put to the school environment. In 2016, the government of Malta enacted the "Healthy Lifestyle Promotion and Care of Non-Communicable Diseases Act," which aimed to promote physical activity and balanced diets to achieve healthy lifestyles and reduce the noncommunicable diseases in all age groups. An intersectoral Advisory Council was set up, and one of its major initiatives was outlining a legislative tool for schools: there was a clear need for improving the school environment to help the whole school community to adopt healthier dietary patterns and lifestyle. The consumption of healthy foods and restrictions on products high in salt, sugar, and fats were encouraged, following nutritional criteria based on the WHO nutrient profiling model and carrying random inspections by specifically trained health practitioners.

In August 2018, the Maltese government issued subsidiary legislation to regulate the food being sold and provided by schools, implement programs for healthy eating, ban advertising or sponsorship of unhealthy foods, and ensure the provision of drinking water in schools. One of the divergences identified across EU states was in planning food procurement tenders for schools that promoted healthy eating and to allow their smooth implementation. It has been important to set clear specifications, with support from the Joint Research Centre and experts [24].

4.3 Poland

In Poland, a 2016 Regulation by the Minister of Health addressed groups of food intended for sale to children and adolescents in the education system. Besides, the School Program Strategy 2017/18–2022/23 has, as one of its goals, the promotion of a healthy, balanced diet among children and parents. In particular, it aims to change the eating habits of children by increasing the share of fruit and vegetables and the intake of milk. In Poland, the food industry is one of the most influential lobby groups, with well-organized representation and significant financial resources. Poland is also one of the participating countries in the Choices Program, an initiative introduced in the Netherlands in 2006 in response to WHO's call for the food industry to take an active voluntary role in tackling obesity. To reduce the consumption of salt, there has been an important consumer awareness initiative through media, schools, and health-care facilities, as well as 16% of salt reduction in bread by 2012. Concerning physical activity, it is mandatory in primary and secondary schools, and it is included in general teaching training [25].

4.4 United Kingdom (UK)

In some countries, reducing childhood obesity is a task shared by the Ministry of Health with the Ministry of Finance (responsible for taxes on food high in saturated fat and sugary soft drinks), the Ministry of Education (for school curricula, healthy nutrition education, and physical activity), and the Ministry of Agriculture and Food Industry (for free school fruit and vegetable schemes and sustainable healthy food supplies) [24]. This is the case of England, opposed to the approach of the Republic of Moldova, where a lack of multisectoral collaboration has been found. The UK Childhood Obesity Plan introduces for the first time a soft drink industry levy and the revenue will be invested in programs to reduce obesity and encourage physical activity, in addition to substantial restrictions for sailing and promoting high sugars and fat drinks or snacks, after the introduction of a tax on sugary drinks was announced in March 2016 and came into force in April 2018.

In some countries, television (TV), radio, and Internet services are regulated with some set standards for advertising to protect children from the overconsumption of unhealthy foods, and this is the case of England, where, the National Office of Communications since 2006, does not allow TV advertisements for such foods to be shown during or close to children TV programs. They also launched a sugar reduction program intending to remove sugar from the food's children frequently eat, paying attention that it is followed by a calorie restriction and not by compensation with extra fats. Also, supporting agricultural innovation by bringing together food business and researchers is part of the project. Support is also given to disadvantaged families, with the distribution of 60 million worth of vouchers that can be exchanged for fresh fruit and vegetables or vitamins. Of course, also physical activity is considered, and it is included in each day at school for at least 30 minutes. It should also be taken into consideration the GREAT commitment of the UK Government in enabling health professionals to support families' diet, as well as training them to face eating behaviors changes and promoting wellbeing [26].

4.5 Moldova

Concerning Moldova, concrete actions to face childhood obesity were only undertaken in 2012. The National Health Policy (2007–2021) was the first policy document that addressed obesity as a priority, involving the society and government, but it was in 2014 when the Moldovan government endorsed the first National Food and Nutrition Program for 2014–2020 and the Action Plan for 2014–2016, with the specific objective to halt the rise of obesity prevalence among children and adults. The 31 July 2007, the Ministry of Health Decision forbids the marketing of energy-dense food with high-fat content and reduced nutritional value in institutions for children. In 2009, new laws prohibited marketing pressure on children to consume healthy drinks. After the Food Law was amended, selling and distribution of unhealthy food within 100 m by schools were banned. The Republic of Moldova became part of COSI from 2013 and participated in the third and fourth rounds of this initiative. Further in 2014, the government adopted the first National Food and Nutrition Programmed for 2014–2020 (NFNP) and its Action Plan with the aim of zero increase in obesity prevalence, employing compulsory nutritional labeling, limitations on advertising, together with the elimination of trans-fats and reduction of sugar and salt [24].

4.6 France

EPODE, or Ensemble, Prévenons L'Obésité Des Enfants (Together, Let us Prevent Childhood Obesity) was established in January 2004, based on the guidelines from the National Health Program recommendations. This program was developed based on the effectiveness observed from the Fleurbaix-Laventie Ville Santé Study, which started in 1992 and continuing, which showed a decrease in childhood obesity rate after the nutritional and physical activity initiatives were implemented in the two towns. The project is supported by the French Ministry of Health, in collaboration with more than five other Ministry, the French National Academy of Medicine, together with some partners like Nestle and Ferrero, financing half of the costs of the program. EPODE now extends to nearly 1.8 million inhabitants in 167 French cities, 20 cities in Spain, and eight cities in Belgium. The project aims to reduce BMI in overweight or obese children promoting physical activity and a healthy diet through three major steps: (1) informing community and families about the obesity problem, using meetings and brochures; (2) Training participants (teachers and professionals); (3) starting the action in schools, distributing educational materials, improving school catering, and hosting food workshop [27].

4.7 Germany

Understanding the importance of obesity as a health issue, and recognizing the worrying increase of overweight adolescences, a range of federal policies were established in Germany to face the issue since, public health services in Germany have played a great role in putting obesity on the political agenda, and they focused on dealing with obesity from child and adolescent health services perspective. The Robert Koch Institute has launched the German Health Interview and Examination Survey for Children and Adolescents (KiGGS-Study), with a baseline study in 2003–2006 and a follow-up study in 2014–2017. The results of the second study were published in March 2018. They pointed to a strong social gradient, with the prevalence of overweight reaching 27.0% and 24.2% in girls and boys respectively, aged 3–17 years with low socioeconomic status compared to 6.5% in girls and 8.9% in boys with high socioeconomic status.

Some of the other vital initiatives in response to the Survey are the National Cycling Plan 2020, which promotes cycling, walking, and the use of public transport and the two programs of the Federal Centre for Health Education (FCHE): Gut Drauf (Feeling Well), which aims to improve the health of children and adolescents aged 12–18 years, and Tutmirgut (Good For Me), aimed at children aged 5-11 years. In 2007, there were 708 programs for overweight or obese children and adolescents in Germany, reaching approximately 44,000 persons [24]. In Germany, policies are implementing a salt reduction in bread and many consumer awareness initiatives regarding a healthy lifestyle, promoted in schools, and via media and Internet [28].

4.8 Denmark

The Danish National Action Plan against Obesity was written to improve awareness in the Danish population and generally reduce high BMI. Children and adolescents are one of their main targets. Concerning nutrition, the aim concerning children's diet is to reduce the number of subjects who consume more energy from fat and sugar and, at the same time, pay attention to the correct fiber intake. Also, life outside the home was provided with healthy food, and parents were supported in taking proper diet choices. Of course, also physical activity is considered, and new guidelines were established, increasing the hours to it dedicated to schools and strengthening the competences of teachers. Suitable playground and outdoor areas were provided, as well as car-free areas near schools and safe foot and cycle paths [29].

5. Conclusion

Handling childhood obesity is undoubtedly challenging despite the substantial progress made concerning healthy nutrition, early life, and increased physical activity. It has also been essential to restrict advertising on TV actively. Still, it should also be taken into consideration to control video games, mobile phones, tablets, and social media since, nowadays, there is no more efficient way to address kids than getting in touch with them through the Internet. Monitoring childhood obesity is, for sure, more rewarding if compared to adults but, initially, for the complexity of relating to young subjects, it can be very onerous.

Consequently and taking into account the role played by multinational food industries in supporting French policies should be considered to further involve in obesity control plans, food, and sports industries. Doing so will make it possible to boost the research resources and, at the same time, allow the markets' sectors, that would possibly be affected by the latest policies and guidelines, to adapt their selling to the new consumer type. It should also be mentioned that some European countries are still not facing the childhood obesity problem, primarily due to inadequate resources and a lack of interface between the health institutions and industries.

In Malta, for example, the requirement of precise definitions for food procurement that tenders on how to set a healthy meal plan in schools was given by the Advisory Council with the support from the EU Joint Research Centre, a proper example of a strategy controlling balance and micronutrient intake of at least one meal per day of all school kids. This strategy, together with the Healthy Weight for Life strategy for 2012–2020 and the Food and Nutrition Policy and Action Plan for Malta 2015–2020, makes Malta one of the most committed European countries in the battle against childhood obesity. The Maltese case is one of the first to be taken into consideration when evaluating the situation.

Conflict of interest

The authors declare no conflict of interest.

Author details

Giulio Nittari[1*], Stefania Scuri[2], Getu Gamo Sagaro[1], Fabio Petrelli[2] and Iolanda Grappasonni[2]

1 Telemedicine and Telepharmacy Centre, University of Camerino, Italy

2 School of Pharmacy, University of Camerino, Italy

*Address all correspondence to: giulio.nittari@unicam.it

IntechOpen

© 2020 The Author(s). Licensee IntechOpen. This chapter is distributed under the terms of the Creative Commons Attribution License (http://creativecommons.org/licenses/by/3.0), which permits unrestricted use, distribution, and reproduction in any medium, provided the original work is properly cited.

References

[1] WHO | Childhood Overweight and Obesity. Available from: https://www.who.int/dietphysicalactivity/childhood/en/ [Accessed: 24 June 2020]

[2] Poskitt EME. Obesity: Childhood obesity. Encyclopedia of Human Nutrition. 2012;**3-4**(14):336-342. DOI: 10.1016/B978-0-12-375083-9.00209-9

[3] WHO. Obesity and Overweight. Available from: https://www.who.int/news-room/fact-sheets/detail/obesity-and-overweight [Accessed: 24 June 2020]

[4] World Health Organization. Resolutions and Decisions, Sixty-Sixth World Health Assembly. WHA66/2013/REC/1. Geneva [Online]. 2013. Available from: https://apps.who.int/gb/ebwha/pdf_files/WHA66-REC1/WHA66_2013_REC1_complete.pdf

[5] Rogers R et al. The relationship between childhood obesity, low socioeconomic status, and race/ethnicity: Lessons from Massachusetts. Childhood Obesity. 2015;**11**(6):691-695. DOI: 10.1089/chi.2015.0029

[6] Nittari G, Scuri S, Petrelli F, Pirillo I, Di Luca NM, Grappasonni I. Fighting obesity in children from European world health organization member states. Epidemiological data, medical-social aspects, and prevention programs. La Clinica Terapeutica. 2019;**170**(3):E223-E230. DOI: 10.7417/CT.2019.2137

[7] World Health Organization. COSI: Severe Obesity among Children Aged 6-9 Years [Online]. 2019. Available from: http://www.euro.who.int/__data/assets/pdf_file/0019/400654/COSI-Severe-Obesity-FS-ENG-LowRes.pdf?ua=1

[8] Spinelli A et al. Prevalence of severe obesity among primary school children in 21 European countries. Obesity Facts. 2019;**12**(2):244-258. DOI: 10.1159/000500436

[9] Cohen AK, Rai M, Rehkopf DH, Abrams B. Educational attainment and obesity: A systematic review. Obesity Reviews. 2013;**14**(12):989-1005. DOI: 10.1111/obr.12062

[10] Kumar S, Kelly AS. Review of childhood obesity: From epidemiology, etiology, and comorbidities to clinical assessment and treatment. Mayo Clinic Proceedings. 2017;**92**(2):251-265. DOI: 10.1016/j.mayocp.2016.09.017

[11] World Health Organization. WHO European Childhood Obesity Surveillance Initiative (COSI). Copenhagen, Denmark: World Health Organization Regional Office for Europe; 2020. [Accessed: 14 September 2020]. Available from: https://www.euro.who.int/en/health-topics/disease prevention/nutrition/activities/who-european-childhood-obesity-surveillance-initiative-cosi

[12] WHO. WHO European childhood obesity surveillance initiative: Overweight and obesity among 6-9-year-old children. Report of the third round of data collection 2012-2013 (2018); 2018

[13] European Commission. EU Action Plan on Childhood Obesity 2014-2020. European Journal of Commission. 2014;(July):68. DOI: 10.2785/36105

[14] WHO. Latest Data Shows Southern European Countries Have Highest Rate of Childhood Obesity. 2018

[15] Lobstein T et al. Child and adolescent obesity: Part of a bigger picture. Lancet. 2015;**385**(9986):2510-2520. DOI: 10.1016/S0140-6736(14)61746-3

[16] World Health Organization. Mapping the health system response to childhood obesity in the WHO European Region An overview and

country perspectives. Copenhagen, Denmark: WHO Regional Office for Europe; 2019. [Accessed: 14 September 2020]. Available from: http://www.euro.who.int/pubrequest

[17] WHO. Global Health Observatory, World Health Organization. Available from: https://www.who.int/data/gho [Accessed: 16 July 2020]

[18] World Health Organization||Food and Agriculture Organization of the United Nations. In: Strengthening nutrition action: A resource guide for countries based on the policy recommendations of the Second International Conference on Nutrition (ICN2). Geneva, Switzerland: World Health Organization; 2018. Available from: https://apps.who.int/iris/handle/10665/274739

[19] World Health Organization. WHO Global Action Plan for the Prevention and Control of NCDs 2013-2020. Geneva, Switzerland: World Health Organization. [Accessed: 14 September 2020]. Available from: https://www.who.int/nmh/events/ncd_action_plan/en/

[20] World Health Organization. Tackling NCDs: "best Buys" and Other Recommended Interventions for the Prevention and Control of Noncommunicable Diseases. Geneva, Switzerland; World Health Organization: 2017. Available from: https://apps.who.int/iris/handle/10665/259232

[21] Joint FAO/WHO evaluation of the work of the Codex Alimentarius Commission. 2003

[22] EU Action Plan on Childhood Obesity 2014-2020 [Online]. Available from: http://www.who.int/dietphysicalactivity/childhood_consequences/en [Accessed: 16 July 2020]

[23] World Health Organization. WHO Report of the Commission on Ending Childhood Obesity: Implementation plan: executive summary. Geneva, Switzerland: World Health Organization. 2016. [Accessed: 14 September 2020]. Available from: https://www.who.int/end-childhood-obesity/publications/echo-plan-executive-summary/en/

[24] World Health Organization. European observatory on health systems and policies: Digital health systems. Eurohealth (Lond). 2019;**25**(1) [Online]. Available from: https://apps.who.int/iris/handle/10665/326127

[25] WHO and Regional Office for Europe. Nutrition, Physical Activity and Obesity Poland [Online]. 2013. Available from: http://www.euro.who.int/en/nutrition-country-profiles [Accessed: 18 July 2020]

[26] Childhood Obesity: Applying All Our Health–GOV.UK. 2020. Available from: https://www.gov.uk/government/publications/childhood-obesity-applying-all-our-health/childhood-obesity-applying-all-our-health [Accessed: 18 July 2020]

[27] EPODE Tackles Childhood Obesity in France | CYP Now. 2019. Available from: https://www.cypnow.co.uk/best-practice/article/epode-tackles-childhood-obesity-in-france [Accessed: 18 July 2020]

[28] World Health Organization and Regional Office for Europe. Nutrition, Physical Activity and Obesity Germany [Online]. 2013. Available from: http://www.euro.who.int/en/nutrition-country-profiles [Accessed: 18 July 2020]

[29] National Board of Health. Center for Health Promotion and Prevention National Action Plan against Obesity [Online]. 2003. Available from: https://www.sst.dk/~/media/681E3288F0A14C2EAA71ED9C4866D01F.ashx

Chapter 11

Unmet Supportive Care Needs of General Cancer

Ezaddin Kamal Mahmod and Saadia Ahmed Khuder

Abstract

Purpose Aside from their oncology condition, cancer patients often experience many ancillary problems, including negative physical symptoms, social isolation, spiritual suffering, and often psychological distress. Supportive care services can be defined as services designed to help patients, their families, and caregivers with their experiences during the diagnosis, treatment, follow-up, and palliative stages of the cancer journey. In an extensive review of the literature, we identified no previous studies that have investigated the SCNs of cancer patients in Iraq or any other Middle Eastern countries. Therefore, this study aims to determine the SCNs of cancer patients in Iraq. Methods The present cross-sectional study and data was conducted in Rezgary teaching and Nankaly Oncology Hospital in the Kurdistan Federal Region of Iraq. A total of 300 eligible cancer patients were invited to participate in the study from February to August, 2018. Eligibility criteria included: 18 years or above; having a definite diagnosis of any type of cancer; physically or mentally able to participate in the study; and being aware of exact diagnosis for at least three months. Results In 15 items of the SCNs, more than 60% of the participants reported that their needs were unmet. Most frequently, unmet needs were related to health system and information, physical and daily living, psychological, and patient care and support domains, and most met needs were related to physical and daily activity domains. Conclusions Kurdish cancer patients had many unmet needs and there is a need for establishing additional supportive care services and educational programs to increase quality of life in Kurdistan Region- Iraq.

Keywords: unmet, cancer patient, supportive care needs, Kurdistan region

1. Introduction

Cancer is the second leading cause of death worldwide, with an estimated global health burden of 193.6 million disability-adjusted life years. This presents a particular challenge for developing nations, which face additional challenges in delivering complex cancer treatments [1]. As a result, the diagnosis of cancer may be experienced as a stressful event that negatively impacts many aspects of patients' lives [2].

After the Iraqi regime change in 2003, rapid changes occurred in the lifestyles of Kurdish people that affected patterns and rates of cancer trends in Kurdistan. Additionally, the population suffers from the cumulative impacts of three vicious wars in Iraq, including targeted genocide against the Kurds and the use of chemical weapons, creating long-term environmental pollution and increasing cancer incidence, aside from their immediate casualties, with especially high rates of hematological malignancies. Tentative published data evidences the increasing cancer prevalence in Kurdistan, [3–6] but related phenomena and care needs have not been explored in detail. This study presents new and more accurate data on the patterns of cancers in Kurdistan and the care needs of cancer patients.

Aside from their oncological condition, spiritual suffering, social isolation, and negative physical and psychological symptoms are among many other problems that cancer patients may experience [7, 8]. Due to this, a variety of supportive care services is needed and has to be reinforced [2, 9]. Such services can be directed to support patients, their families, and caregivers during different stages of the cancer journey, such as at the initial post-diagnosis phase, the duration of treatment and follow-up, and even end of life care [6]. Currently, offering supportive care services is regarded to be of equal importance to the diagnosis and treatment of cancer itself, and it involves more holistic healthcare provision compared to the biomedical approach that dominates mainstream oncology treatment [10]. The first step in planning any supportive care services for cancer patients is identifying their supportive care needs (SCNs) [1, 11, 12].

While several studies have investigated the SCNs of cancer patients worldwide, most were conducted in Western countries [11, 13–20]. Few studies have investigated the SCNs of cancer patients in non-Western settings, but pioneering research indicates that cancer patients in the latter have many unmet supportive needs, albeit there are numerous methodological issues and diverse findings between studies in Western and non-Western countries [21–25].

Unmet needs are defined as "the requirement for some desirable, necessary or useful action to be taken or some resource to be provided in order for the person to attain optimal well-being" [26, 27]. A systematic review by Harrison et al. [28] concluded that unmet needs were frequently reported in relation to activities of daily living, psychological and psychosocial issues, the need for information, and physical concerns. Similar findings were reported by Fiszer et al. [29].

SCNs are a "culture-dependent" notion. Thus, cultural issues must be taken into consideration when developing an effective supportive care program [23]. After an extensive literature review, no previous studies found to investigate the SCNs of cancer patients in Iraq or in any other Middle Eastern countries. Hence, this study aimed to determine the SCNs of cancer patients in Iraq.

2. Materials and methods

This study was conducted in Rezgary Teaching Hospital and Nankaly Oncology Hospital in the Kurdistan Federal Region of Iraq. Both hospitals are educational centers affiliated with Hawler Medical University, a referral center for sub-special cancer treatment.

A total of 300 eligible cancer patients were invited to participate in the study from February to August, 2018. Participant eligibility criteria included being aged 18 years or above; having a definite diagnosis of any type of cancer; being physically or mentally able to participate in the study; and being aware of exact diagnosis for at least three months.

Participants completed a questionnaire comprising two parts. Participants' basic socio-demographic and disease-related characteristics were assessed in the first part. In addition, information regarding medical treatments was obtained from the participants' health records. The second part consisted of an SCNs Survey (SCNS), used to examine the SCNs of cancer patients; it is derived from previous studies [30]. The SCNS comprises 48 items addressing five domains of needs:

- H&I: health system and information (15 items).
- NS: non-specific items (4 items).
- P&D: physical and daily living (7 items).
- P&S: patient care and support (8 items).
- Psycho: psychological (11 items).
- Sex: sexuality (3 items).

Each item was based on a five-point Likert scale (1 = not applicable or no need, 2 = satisfied, 3 = low need, 4 = moderate need, 5 = high need). To determine the SCN score, the five-point Likert scale was dichotomized to unmet need (for moderate need or high need) or no need (for not applicable, satisfied, or low need). Previous researches have used this scoring system widely [23, 24].

The English version of the SCN SF48 was translated into Kurdish by two independent English-Kurdish translators. Eight academic staff at Hawler Medical University (HMU) College of Nursing reviewed the questionnaire to ensure face and content validity. Based on their comments, minor amendments were made. The internal reliability coefficients (Cronbach's alpha values) of the translated questionnaire were substantial (greater than 0.90) when piloted with 25 cancer patients.

The participants were recruited from inpatient wards of both studied hospitals. Participants were provided with information about the study and the questionnaire to fill in. If participants were incapable to complete the questionnaire due to literacy problems, the researchers assisted them to complete it with a short interview.

Many cancer patients in Iraq may not know the exact diagnosis of their disease, and only limited information is disclosed to them, as highlighted in previous research. Consequently, an important clinical concern in this study was to determine participants' own awareness of their diagnosis of cancer [3–6]. In order to identify this and prevent unwanted revelations, this information was obtained from the patients' caregivers and/or healthcare professionals and then checked with the patients through a short private interview. This procedure was approved by the Regional Ethics Committee at HMU College of Nursing. All participants were informed of the study aims and objectives, and informed consent was obtained. Participants were told that participation was entirely voluntary, and their decision would not affect their care or statutory rights. They were also assured of data anonymity and their right to withdraw from the study at any time.

Data analysis was performed using SPSS version 22 (SPSS Inc., Chicago, Illinois). Analyzing the demographic characteristics, cancer-related information, and unmet and met SCNs of participants was undertaken using descriptive statistics (frequency, percentage, mean, and standard deviation).

3. Results

Participants' demographic and cancer-related features are reported in **Table 1**. Most of the participants were female (66.7%), married (84.7%), educated at primary level (19.7%), employed as independent workers (65.7%), and living in urban areas (54.7%). More than half of them were aged above 48 years old. The particular cancer

No.	Variable	Categories	N	%
1	Age group	18–27 years	26	8.7
		28–37 years	35	11.7
		38–47 years	58	19.3
		48–57 years	76	25.3
		58–67 years	72	24.0
		68–77 years	28	9.3
		78–87 years	5	1.7
2	Gender	Male	100	33.3
		Female	200	66.7
3	Living situation	Urban	164	54.7
		Rural	136	45.3
4	Marital status	Married	254	84.7
		Single	43	14.3
		Widowed	1	0.3
		Divorced	2	0.7
5	Education status	Illiterate	129	43.0
		Read and write	37	12.3
		Primary school	59	19.7
		High school graduate	50	16.7
		College and postgraduate	25	8.3
6	Occupational status	Student	12	4.0
		Employed	51	17.0
		Unemployed	21	7.0
		Independent worker	197	65.7
		Retired	19	6.3
7	Cancer origin	Breast cancer	120	40.0
		Colon cancer	28	9.3
		Leukemia	11	3.6
		Myeloma	1	0.3
		Non-Hodgkin's lymphoma	6	2.0
		Ovarian cancer	23	7.7
		Pancreatic cancer	4	1.3
		Prostate cancer	10	3.3
		Lung cancer	34	11.3
		Rectal cancer	2	0.7
		Uterine cancer	2	0.7
		Other	60	20.0
8	Type of treatment	Hormonal therapy	54	18.0
		Chemotherapy	253	84.3
		Radiotherapy	86	28.7
		Surgical removal of cancer	134	44.7
		Immunotherapy	104	34.7
		Bone marrow treatment	45	15.0

Table 1.
Participant demographic and disease-related characteristics.

diagnosis, treatment received, and the taking of treatment were noted; over 40% of the 120 patients participating in this study had been diagnosed with breast cancer, and their treatment was primarily chemotherapy and/or radiation therapy. Most of them attended treatment and were receiving chemotherapy.

The data analysis shows that in 13 items of SCNS, more than 65% of the participants reported that their SCNs were not satisfied (**Table 2**). This demonstrates that the participants have many unmet SCNs. In terms of domain, 6 of these 13 items concerned H&I; 3 were Psycho; 2 were in NS; and 1 each was in P&D and the P&S domains. In H&I, three 3 of the most unmet needs were "Being given information (written, diagrams, drawings) about aspects of managing your illness and side-effects at home," "Being informed about your test results as soon as feasible," and "Being adequately informed about the benefits and side-effects of treatments before you choose to have them." These results highlight that the patients have many unmet needs, especially in the information domain. Within the Psycho domain, the 3 most unmet needs were for "Concerns about the worries of those close to you," "Anxiety," and "Concerns about the ability of those close to you to cope with caring for you." This means that the patients were distressed about the outcomes of the disease or worried about the changes in the routines of their disease and their families. The most frequent unmet needs were "Concerns about your financial situation" and "Concerns about getting to and from the hospital," which were related to the non-specific domain. In the P&S domain, only one item was reported as highly unsatisfactory by more than 83% of participants, which was "Lack of energy and tiredness."

Participants' mean scores in the SCNS domains are illustrated in **Table 3**. In four domains (Psycho, H&I, P&D, and P&S), the participants gained scores of more than 10, which indicates that most of the participants had many unmet needs. However, only the sexuality domain had a score of less than 10. The most unmet needs were for the domains of H&I (36.42), P&D (35.56), Psycho (28.4), P&S (14.27), sexuality (7.76) and non-specific (6.07).

Items	Domain	No.	%
Lack of energy and tiredness	P&D	251	83.7
Concerns about the worries of those close to you	Psycho	249	83
Being given information (written, diagrams, drawings) about aspects of managing your illness and side-effects at home	H&I	249	83.0
Being informed about your test results as soon as feasible	H&I	244	81.3
Being adequately informed about the benefits and side-effects of treatments before you choose to have them	H&I	241	80.3
Concerns about the ability of those close to you to cope with caring for you	Psycho	232	77.3
Being informed about cancer which is under control or diminishing	H&I	231	77.0
Being informed about things you can do to help yourself get well	H&I	224	74.7
Having access to professional counseling (e.g., psychologist, social worker, counselor, nurse specialist) if you/your family/friends need it	H&I	223	74.3
Concerns about your financial situation	NS	211	70.3
Concerns about getting to and from the hospital	NS	209	69.7
Anxiety	Psycho	202	67.3
Family or friends being allowed with you in hospital whenever you want	P&S	197	65.7

Table 2.
Top 15 unmet SCNs of cancer patients.

Domain	Mean	Std. Deviation
Health system and information	36.42	8.15
Non-specific	6.07	2.11
Patient care and support	14.27	4.68
Physical and daily activity	35.56	9.50
Psychological	28.4	7.98
Sexuality	7.72	3.36

Table 3.
The score of participants in each domain on SCNs survey.

Items	Domain	No.	(%)
Itching	P&D	253	84.3
Being treated like a person, not just another case	H&I	252	84
Keeping a positive outlook	Psycho	233	77.7
Nausea and vomiting	P&D	219	73.0
Swelling of arms, legs, or abdomen	P&D	217	72.3
Being treated in a hospital or clinic that is as physically pleasant as possible	H&I	204	68
Learning to feel in control of your situation	Psycho	203	67.7
Having one member of hospital staff with whom you can talk about all aspects of your condition, treatment, and follow-up	H&I	198	66
Feelings about death and dying	Psycho	195	65
Prickling or numb sensation	P&D	185	61.7

Table 4.
Top 10 most frequently met needs of participants.

The 10 most frequently met needs of participants are reported in **Table 4**. More than 70% of the participants reported that they have no needs in these items. As shown in this table, in terms of the studied domains, 4 of the commonly met needs related to aspects of physical and daily activity; and 3 each related to the H&I domain. Interestingly, 4 of these items are related to P&D (3 items) and H&I mean no need to help in physically and patients have equal rights to being treatment and follow-up.

4. Discussion

To our knowledge, this is the first study that has investigated the SCNs of cancer patients in the Kurdistan Federal Region, and indeed Iraq in general. The results demonstrate that Kurdish cancer patients have many unmet SCNs, especially in the domains of health system, information, P&D. Most of the participants reported unmet SCNs in 13 items of SCNs.

In an extensive review of the literature, it was found that some studies reported that cancer patients have low needs; [11, 19] but most studies highlight that cancer patients in both non-Western [17–21] and Western countries [9, 14, 31] have many SCNs. None of the analyzed studies reported such high levels of needs as reported by the participants of our study.

The results of our study demonstrate that 6 out of 15 most frequently unmet SCNs of cancer patients are related to the H&I domain. This finding is to some degree different with previous studies conducted in Western countries, which reported the H&I domain to be the second or third domain in which cancer patients' needs are unmet [6, 9, 13, 32–36]. Conversely, the findings of other studies conducted in Southwest Asia indicated that H&I domain needs are among the most frequent unmet SCNs of cancer patients [17, 20, 21, 34]. Likewise, a comparative study revealed that Hong Kong breast cancer patients ranked H&I needs as the most frequent unmet SCNs, while German women consider needs from P&D and Psycho needs to be the most frequently unmet supportive care they experienced [19]. Therefore, this finding supports that SCNs are a culture-dependent issue [19]. Additionally, survivors' needs are dynamic and might change over time. A shift in perceived cancer survivors' needs from informational needs to Psycho needs has been found by researchers, partly attributable to improvements in information delivery over the years [37]. Further research is required to ascertain whether the predominance of H&I needs in the Kurdistan region can be justified by reasons like changing expectations for information provision due to ease of access to internet-based information, or an institutional deficit instigated by other possible reasons, such as lacking clinical resources or insufficient staff education. No additional evidence could be established on the prevalence of cancer patients' informational needs, and whether these needs have changed over time or been influenced by contemporary changes in information seeking practices.

The results of our study also indicated that Psycho needs are the second category of unmet SCNs of Kurdish cancer patients, after H&I needs. This finding is consistent with the results of other studies in non-Western countries [17, 20, 21, 37]. It should be noted that Kurdish cancer patients are often unaware of the prognosis of their diseases, and consider cancer to be a conventional, curable disease. Consequently, it can be inferred that the nondisclosure of cancer prognosis for most Kurdish cancer patients may explain the unusually low level of Psycho SCNs found among Kurdish cancer patients.

The results of this study have important clinical implications, particularly in demonstrating that cancer patients in the Kurdistan Region of Iraq have many SCNs in different domains. Few established supportive care programs are available for patients with cancer in Iraq, and our findings underline that there is an urgent need for such programs to be established. Most unmet SCNs cancer patients in Iraq are from the perspective of the domains of H&I and P&D. Thus, educating cancer patients and meeting their H&I and Psycho needs should be considered as a fundamental part of supportive care programs.

There are limitations to our study. This study was conducted in two oncology centers in the Kurdistan Region of Iraq; even though the setting comprises the main referral center for a large province in northern of Iraq, it does not include all areas of Iraq. The findings related to non-specific SCNs ought to be interpreted with caution, considering the taboo associated with sexual issues in Iraq and Kurdish culture. Further studies are necessary that investigate the SCNs of different cultures in the Middle East. Using other data collection methods, including private interviews, may increase the validity of results in the sexual domain of SCNs.

5. Conclusion

This study highlights that Kurdish cancer patients have many unmet needs in all domains of SCNs. These findings indicate that programs and services to address the SCNs are urgently needed. Future research in Iraq should shed light on the particular SCNs of patients in cultural contexts, to help tailor more comprehensive and holistic care, particularly for cancer patients, in order to improve the quality of healthcare services provided.

Ethical considerations

The research project was approved by the Ethics Committee of Hawler Medical University, College of Nursing (Project No. 3, approval date: 2016/03/16).

Author details

Ezaddin Kamal Mahmod* and Saadia Ahmed Khuder
Hawler Medical University, College of Nursing and Midwifery,
Erbil City, Kurdistan Region, Iraq

*Address all correspondence to: ezaddinbotany@yahoo.com

IntechOpen

© 2021 The Author(s). Licensee IntechOpen. This chapter is distributed under the terms of the Creative Commons Attribution License (http://creativecommons.org/licenses/by/3.0), which permits unrestricted use, distribution, and reproduction in any medium, provided the original work is properly cited.

References

[1] Global Burden of Disease Cancer Collaboration, Fitzmaurice C, Dicker D, Pain A, Hamavid H, Moradi-Lakeh M, et al. The Global Burden of Cancer 2013. JAMA Oncol 2015; 1:505-527.

[2] Carey M, Lambert S, Smits R, Paul C, Sanson-Fisher R, Clinton-McHarg T. The unfulfi lled promise: A systematic review of interventions to reduce the unmet supportive care needs of cancer patients. Support Care Cancer 2012; 20:207-219.

[3] Khoshnaw N, Francis B, Safar B, et al (2014) Cytogenetic response in chronic myeloid leukaemia patients treated with imatinib mesylate homolog-drugs: 6 year's transitional study. J Cancer Therapy, 5,453-459.

[4] Majid R, Mohammed H, Hassan H, et al (2012). A populationbased study of Kurdish breast cancer in northern Iraq: Hormone receptor and HER2 status. A comparison with Arabic women and United States SEER data. BMC Women's Health, 12, 16.

[5] Zangana A, Garota S (2012). Risk factors of breast cancer in a sample of Kurdish women of Kurdistan Region - Iraq: a comparative study between pre-menopausal and postmenopausal women, Zanco. J Med Sci, 16,3.

[6] Othman RT, Abdulljabar R, Saeed A, et al (2011). Cancer incidence rates in the Kurdistan region/Iraq from 2007-2009. Asian Pac J Cancer Prev, 12, 1261-1264.

[7] Fujisawa D, Park S, Kimura R, Suyama I, Koyama Y, Takeuchi M, et al. Unmet supportive needs of cancer patients in an acute care hospital in Japan--a census study. Support Care Cancer 2010;18:1393-1403.

[8] Stiefel F, Guex P. Palliative and supportive care: At the frontier of medical omnipotence. Ann Oncol 1996; 7:135-138.

[9] Johnston G, Vukic A, Parker S. Cultural understanding in the provision of supportive and palliative care: Perspectives in relation to an indigenous population. BMJ Support Palliat Care 2013;3:61-68.

[10] Fincham L, Copp G, Caldwell K, Jones L, Tookman A. Supportive care: Experiences of cancer patients. Eur J Oncol Nurs 2005; 9:258-268.

[11] Whelan TJ, Mohide EA, Willan AR, Arnold A, Tew M, Sellick S, et al. The supportive care needs of newly diagnosed cancer patients attending a regional cancer center. Cancer 1997;80:1518-1524.

[12] Jones R, Regan M, Ristevski E, Breen S. Patients' perception of communication with clinicians during screening and discussion of cancer supportive care needs. Patient Educ Couns 2011; 85:209-215.

[13] Beesley VL, Price MA, Webb PM, O'Rourke P, Marquart L, Butow PN, Australian Ovarian Cancer Study Group, Australian Ovarian Cancer Study-Quality of Life Study Investigators. Changes in supportive care needs after fi rst-line treatment for ovarian cancer: Identifying care priorities and risk factors for future unmet needs. Psychooncology 2013; 22:1565-1571.

[14] Bender JL, Wiljer D, To MJ, Bedard PL, Chung P, Jewett MA, et al. Testicular cancer survivors' supportive care needs and use of online support: A cross-sectional survey. Support Care Cancer 2012; 20:2737-2746.

[15] Chambers SK, Girgis A, Occhipinti S, Hutchison S, Turner J, Morris B, et al. Psychological distress and unmet supportive care needs in cancer patients and carers who contact cancer helplines. Eur J Cancer Care Engl 2012;21:213-223.

[16] Janda M, Steginga S, Dunn J, Langbecker D, Walker D, Eakin E. Unmet supportive care needs and interest in services among patients with a brain tumour and their carers. Patient Educ Couns 2008; 71:251-258.

[17] Rainbird K, Perkins J, Sanson-Fisher R, Rolfe I, Anseline P. The needs of patients with advanced, incurable cancer. Br J Cancer 2009;101:759-764.

[18] Smith DP, Supramaniam R, King MT, Ward J, Berry M, Armstrong BK. Age, health, and education determine supportive care needs of men younger than 70 years with prostate cancer. J Clin Oncol 2007;25:2560-2566.

[19] Snyder CF, Garrett-Mayer E, Blackford AL, Brahmer JR, Carducci MA, Pili R, et al. Concordance of cancer patients' function, symptoms, and supportive care needs. Qual Life Res 2009;18:991-998.

[20] Sutherland G, Hill D, Morand M, Pruden M, McLachlan SA. Assessing the unmet supportive care needs of newly diagnosed patients with cancer. Eur J Cancer Care Engl 2009;18:577-584.

[21] Au A, Lam W, Tsang J, Yau TK, Soong I, Yeo W, et al. Supportive care needs in Hong Kong Chinese women confronting advanced breast cancer. Psychooncology 2013; 22:1144-1151.

[22] Chen, S.C., Lai, Y.H., Liao, C.T., Chang, J.T.C., Lin, C.Y., Fan, K.H. and Huang, B.S., 2013. Supportive care needs in newly diagnosed oral cavity cancer patients receiving radiation therapy. Psycho-Oncology, *22*(6), pp.1220-1228.

[23] Lam WW, Au AH, Wong JH, Lehmann C, Koch U, Fielding R, et al. Unmet supportive care needs: A cross-cultural comparison between Hong Kong Chinese and German Caucasian women with breast cancer. Breast Cancer Res Treat 2011; 130:531-541.

[24] Liao YC, Liao WY, Shun SC, Yu CJ, Yang PC, Lai YH. Symptoms, psychological distress, and supportive care needs in lung cancer patients. Support Care Cancer 2011; 19:1743-1751.

[25] Okuyama T, Akechi T, Yamashita H, Toyama T, Nakaguchi T, Uchida M, et al. Oncologists' recognition of supportive care needs and symptoms of their patients in a breast cancer outpatient consultation. Jpn J Clin Oncol 2011; 41:1251-1258.

[26] Lattimore-Foot GG. Needs Assessment in Tertiary and Secondary Oncology Practice: A Conceptual and Methodological Exposition. University of Newcastle; 1996.

[27] Campbell HS, Sanson-Fisher R, Taylor-Brown J, Hayward L, Wang XS, Turner D. The cancer support person's unmet needs survey: Psychometric properties. Cancer 2009; 115:3351-3359.

[28] Harrison JD, Young JM, Price MA, Butow PN, Solomon MJ. What are the unmet supportive care needs of people with cancer? A systematic review. Support Care Cancer 2009;17: 1117-1128.

[29] Fiszer C, Dolbeault S, Sultan S, Brédart A. Prevalence, intensity, and predictors of the supportive care needs of women diagnosed with breast cancer: A systematic review. Psychooncology 2014; 23:361-374.

[30] Bonevski B, Sanson-Fisher R, Girgis A, Burton L, Cook P, Boyes A. Evaluation of an instrument to assess the needs of patients with cancer. Supportive Care Review Group. Cancer 2000; 88:217-225.

[31] Zebrack BJ, Mills J, Weitzman TS. Health and supportive care needs of young adult cancer patients and survivors. J Cancer Surviv 2007; 1:137-145.

[32] Jorgensen ML, Young JM, Harrison JD, Solomon MJ. Unmet supportive care needs in colorectal cancer: Differences by age. Support Care Cancer 2012; 20:1275-1281.

[33] Sanders SL, Bantum EO, Owen JE, Thornton AA, and Stanton AL. Supportive care needs in patients with lung cancer. Psycho oncology 2010; 19:480-489.

[34] Steginga SK, Occhipinti S, Dunn J, Gardiner RA, Heathcote P, Yaxley J. The supportive care needs of men with prostate cancer (2000). Psycho oncology 2001;10:66-75.

[35] Minstrell M, Winzenberg T, Rankin N, Hughes C, Walker J. Supportive care of rural women with breast cancer in Tasmania, Australia: Changing needs over time. Psychooncology 2008; 17:58-65.

[36] McDowell ME, Occhipinti S, Ferguson M, Dunn J, Chambers SK. Predictors of change in unmet supportive care needs in cancer. Psychooncology 2010; 19:508-516.

[37] Sanson-Fisher, R., Girgis, A., Boyes, A., Bonevski, B., Burton, L., Cook, P. and Supportive Care Review Group, 2000. The unmet supportive care needs of patients with cancer. Cancer, 88(1), pp.226-237.